OUTBACK HEROES

OUTBACK HEROES

75 years of the Royal Flying Doctor Service of Australia

Kay Batstone

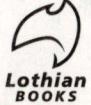

Lothian
BOOKS

Thomas C. Lothian Pty Ltd
132 Albert Road, South Melbourne, 3205
www.lothian.com.au

National Library of Australia
Cataloguing-in-Publication data:

Batstone, Kay.
    Outback heroes : 75 years of the Royal Flying Doctor Service.
    ISBN 0 7344 0575 8.

    1. Royal Flying Doctor Service of Australia - History.
    2. Rural health services - Australia - History.
    3. Aeronautics in medicine - Australia - History.
    I. Title.

362.1042570994

Cover design by Ektavo
Text design by Patrick Cannon
Typeset by Cannon Typesetting in 12/16 Bembo
Printed in Australia by Griffin Press

Note: Every effort has been made to contact the copyright owners
of quoted material. Please contact the publisher if you have any
information regarding this matter.

Foreword

. . . .

'This book salutes the extraordinary seventy-five-year history of the Royal Flying Doctor Service and the extraordinary people who contributed to its creation and continue to carry on its work.'

Indeed!

This is how this remarkable book closes. *Outback Heroes* is a fresh approach to this wonderful story.

Although I have been associated with the Royal Flying Doctor Service for more than forty years, I found in these pages much I did not know. I read it, appropriately, in Broken Hill where a vibrant flying doctor base has existed throughout most of the history of the service. This added to the impact of the tale so vividly portrayed by author Kay Batstone. The story of John Flynn found in these pages is remarkable for it depicts a young man deemed by some as a failure when he was young who, fortuitously or otherwise, when directed into his rightful field knew no bounds. His energy, ideas and enthusiasm were exactly what were required; he liked people and knew how to stimulate them into activity. It was such an infectious process. All the time he was leaving a trail of the most memorable aphorisms, many of which are recorded here. They are still relevant today.

Kay Batstone's *Outback Heroes* illustrates also that wonderful Australian quality of helping others. Thus the development of the Royal Flying Doctor Service saw people, particularly those living in populated regions, helping their less fortunate compatriots struggling in the remote areas of this vast country.

Kay tells many moving stories of resourcefulness, courage, warmth and generosity involving our fellow Australians. The tales and exploits of the nurses and pilots collected together highlight how the Royal Flying Doctor Service is very much a team where no one person is more special than another. In the past some of these people have not featured as greatly as they should. In fact, books could and should be written about engineers, base directors, refuellers, office workers and many others who have contributed in such an important way to the service.

All these good people exist today and will continue to come in the future. They have made, and will continue to make, the Royal Flying Doctor Service uniquely great — and very Australian. Just as ANZAC has something important to do with our national character, so, too, does our Royal Flying Doctor Service.

This is the strong and wonderful message Kay Batstone has so skillfully developed in *Outback Heroes*.

Dr Michael Long AM

Contents

. . . .

Preface

. . . .

This book commemorates the seventy-fifth anniversary of the Royal Flying Doctor Service which took to the air in 1928. However, the genesis of the Service can be traced back to 1911, when the Reverend John Flynn, in his role as outback missionary, began to develop an awareness of the Inlanders' struggle to live and work in the bush with almost non-existent access to medical care. Thereafter, Flynn made it his life's work to deliver Inlanders from their plight by establishing a network of cottage hospitals that evolved into the Flying Doctor Service. The corollary to this endeavour was the creation of a communications system that provided the means whereby the sick or injured could call for help. It was an enormous undertaking and one which richly deserves to be brought to the notice of each new generation of Australians.

In writing this book, I have sought to pay tribute to the outback heroes, past and present, who have been involved with the Flying Doctor Service throughout its long and illustrious history, and before. It is about the people who have delivered this service and about the people who have received it. It is about the living conditions of people who bravely took up the challenge of the outback to create an Australian rural way of life.

There is no more eloquent way to tell this story and to breathe life into an otherwise historical account than to let these people speak for themselves. Accordingly, the book has been written in five sections, each from the perspective of the main protagonists – Flynn himself, Alfred Traeger who developed the famous pedal radio, the aviators, the nurses and the doctors. And throughout we hear the voices of the Inlanders, who embraced the Service and who, seventy-five years later, continue to support it with the same passion.

The medical needs of people in the bush are constantly changing and the demand for the services of the Flying Doctor organisation has never been greater. Each year the number and variety of services increases, as does the number of personnel who deliver them. The challenge for the organisation in the future will be to utilise advanced aviation and medical technology to provide the most up-to-date health services to rural and remote communities. With its well-established infrastructure, the Royal Flying Doctor Service is ideally placed to carry out this role in this new millennium.

Acknowledgments

. . . .

Much of the material describing the early years of the Royal Flying Doctor Service (RFDS) comes from *The Inlander*, a magazine to which the Reverend John Flynn was chief contributor and editor, and which appeared on and off from 1913 to 1929. In it can be traced Flynn's thought processes as he developed his network of cottage hospitals under the auspices of the Australian Inland Mission (AIM) and later formulated the plans for an aerial medical service. Similarly, magazines like the *NSW Presbyterian* and *The Presbyterian Messenger* (journals of the Presbyterian Church) and *Frontier News* (the journal of the AIM) provided a chronicle of both Flynn's experiences and those of the AIM nursing sisters and patrol padres, and the flying doctors when they appeared from 1928. Excerpts from journals of the different sections of the RFDS and interviews with RFDS personnel show the contemporary position.

Two excellent historical accounts, *John Flynn: Apostle to the Inland* by W Scott McPheat (1963) and *The Flying Doctor Story 1928–78* by Michael Page (1977), provided a guide through the mass of data that makes up the story of the history of the RFDS.

Special thanks go to Chris Benaud (Marketing/PR Manager, RFDS, South Eastern Section) for his support throughout this project and for his help in coordinating interviews with personnel from the RFDS. Thanks also to Stephen Penberthy (Public Affairs Manager, RFDS, Queensland Section), and to the following people who took time out of their busy workdays to talk about the RFDS: Dr Don Bowley (Senior Medical Officer), Captain Peter Brooke (Pilot), Jane Bryant (Women's Health Nurse), Leesa Catford (Child and Family Health Nurse), Dr Mike Hill (Senior Medical Officer), John Lynch (CEO Central Operations), Captain Steve McLay (Senior Base Pilot), Susan Markwell (Senior Flight Nurse), Gary Oldman (IT Manager), Noel Passlow (Senior Base Engineer), Dr Anne Wakatama (Chief Medical Officer), David White (Nurse Manager) and Robert Williams (Psychologist).

My thanks also to Gerry Macdonald (Executive Director, Australian Council) and Kerrie Smith for their help in sourcing photographs from the RFDS collection.

FLYNN OF THE INLAND

1

The Man and the Mission

. . . .

As the twenty-first century unfolds we have reached a level of sophistication that allows us to accept fairly readily whatever scientific and technological developments have come our way and, barring ethical considerations, to embrace without awe the prospect of what is to come. This was not the case at the beginning of the twentieth century. Certainly, the public were delighted and intrigued by the progress that had been achieved – telegraph, telephone, film, the motor vehicle – but many were sceptical about what further might be possible. In a world that proceeded in a more leisurely fashion than today, to hasten slowly was desirable. On to this stage strode the unlikely figure of the Reverend John Flynn who announced to a largely disbelieving world his plans for protecting the health and well-being of the people of the Australian Inland. His idea was to service the medical needs of the Inlanders with doctors arriving by aeroplane, landing on airstrips situated in the most inaccessible locations, and summoned by a radio network stretching across the continent. Bearing in mind that aviation at this time was in its infancy, remote airstrips were non-existent and the radio system that Flynn envisaged had yet to be invented, it must have seemed like the stuff of science fiction. But this remarkable man had a vision, and for the rest of his life, would not stray from it. 'For, if we once dream it, the rest is easy.'[1]

The Rev. C Goy, at a memorial service conducted by the General
Assembly of Victoria after Flynn's death, summed it up in this way:
'The secret of his life, quite apart from his keen intellect, his natural
gifts for organisation, his tremendous tenacity of purpose, and his
remarkable manner of enlisting interest and support in his undertaking, was the simple fact that early he found his life's work, and
stayed in it to the end.'[2]

Flynn's interest in people in rural areas began during the years
from 1899 to 1903 when he was a pupil/teacher with the Education
Department of Victoria. Initially he had wanted to become a clergy-
man, an interest stimulated by his family's involvement in the activities
of churches of various denominations over several generations. But
this ambition had been thwarted by the lack of funds available to
undertake a theology course at university. Flynn's father was also a
teacher but not well-off, having had to bear the financial impost of
raising a family of three – Eugene, Rosetta and John – with the help
of paid housekeepers after John's mother died bearing her fifth child.
(Another child had died earlier and the family were to lose Eugene
to tuberculosis at age twenty-three.) Thus did the impecunious John
follow in his father's footsteps as an educator. He taught mainly in
schools in the Melbourne suburbs, except for a six-month stint
in 1901 at a school near Morwell, about 160 kilometres south-east of
Melbourne, where he mixed with the local farming community,
learned to handle a rifle, and found time to explore the surrounding
countryside on a bicycle. Back in Melbourne in 1902 he found much
to occupy his spare time, teaching bible classes, organising social
activities, writing articles for the local paper, enrolling in a first aid
course and developing an interest in photography. His aptitude for
teaching, writing, communicating, photography and administering to
the injured were to be invaluable later in life when he was travelling
and working in the outback and seeking to give the Inlanders a
practical demonstration of his concern for their affairs.

Flynn's teaching job was not well paid and he struggled to put
aside the funds necessary for university fees. But there were other

routes to the ministry. The Presbyterian Church of Victoria ran mission departments catering for those at home and abroad. While seeking to minister to non-Christians overseas, the Church was also mindful of its responsibilities to its flock closer to home. Accordingly the Home Mission Department needed young men to live and work in isolated communities. They were paid a small stipend and, if they pursued their studies, gained entrance to Ormond College at the University of Melbourne, where young men trained for the Presbyterian ministry.

Flynn successfully applied and was appointed in 1903 as a home missionary at Beech Forest, a timber town in the rugged Otway Ranges of southern Victoria. Flynn travelled his parish on horseback, caring for both the physical and spiritual needs of the loggers and timbermen and their families. These were pioneering folk, rough and hard-working but friendly, who appreciated Flynn's quiet manner, his generosity and his practical skills. After eighteen months, Flynn left for his next appointment in Buchan in Gippsland in south-east Victoria, already much wiser in the ways of ministering to an itinerant group in crude circumstances, without the automatic gravitas conferred by formal church halls and buildings. Flynn achieved a degree of notoriety by purchasing a magic lantern and giving slide lectures, using as his subject his developing collection of photos of the district. He completed his Home Mission studies in 1907 and at last became eligible to enrol in theology at Ormond College. He was now a 'mature age' student of twenty-seven. In addition, he became home missionary for the inner city suburb of Montague.

By all accounts Flynn did not cover himself with distinction academically, apparently having particular difficulty with Greek and Hebrew. Given that realising his ultimate ambitions in no way depended on a grasp of ancient languages, he may later have been struck with the irrelevance of his early concern! His studies also suffered by his time and energy being diverted to activities outside of the scope of his course. One such activity was a three-month shearer's mission he undertook at the end of 1909 at the request of the Victorian Director of Home Missions, the Rev. Donald Cameron, who regarded Flynn as a young man with great promise. Travelling by coach, train and motor buggy, Flynn covered the area between Melbourne and Mount Gambier in South Australia. Conscious that many of the shearers had little use for established religion, he related to them by whatever means he sensed would best reach them, whether by religious instruction, first aid lectures, lantern shows, or a combination of all three.

During his tour of duty, he met Hamilton's Presbyterian minister, the Rev. John Andrew Barber, a meeting that was to prove propitious. The two men got along well, with their concern for rural dwellers a common interest. W Scott McPheat, in his meticulously researched book, *John Flynn: Apostle to the Inland*, gives this account of one of their conversations: 'One night when they were discussing literature suitable for bush people, Flynn mentioned a shearer's observation that a copy of a funeral service would have been useful when he recently buried his mate far from a church centre; all he and his friends could do at the graveside was sing Auld Lang Syne. Others had asked him to write out his first aid lectures.'[3]

It struck Flynn as a sad state of affairs that men wishing to give a fallen mate a Christian burial might lack the knowledge by which to do it. Distressing also was the thought that an injured man might suffer needlessly for lack of access to someone with even elementary information about caring for a wound or splinting a broken limb. With these thoughts in mind, Barber and Flynn came up with the idea of *The Bushman's Companion*. The book was to be a practical and spiritual guide, not only covering such things as instruction in first aid and the words of a burial service, but also incorporating hints for the treatment of common ailments, directions for making a will, selections from the scriptures, quotes from poets like Tennyson and Lawson, hymns, prayers, and blank pages for notes, accounts and addresses. (The poignancy of the last is striking. As a bushman went about his solitary outback travels, how many addresses would he actually need to remember?)

Back in Melbourne, Flynn got to work, seeking advice from informed parties about the book's content and raising money for the cost of its production. It emerged in September 1910 and copies of it still exist today in various archives. It was of great importance to its readership – it may well have been the only book the recipients had ever owned, or at least the only book that had ever spoken directly to their needs – and yet it is such a small, unpretentious volume. To hold a copy in the hand is to wonder in whose pocket or saddlebag it has travelled and what comfort and succour it might have brought to its owner.

Flynn began his book with an 'Open Letter to Bushmen' in which he introduced himself and extended the hand of friendship, saying in part:

> Comrades, Some of you will look upon me as not altogether a stranger, although we have met only once; but to you all, known and unknown, let me extend the heartiest of greetings. After all, it is not necessary to have met face to face to feel a sense of comradeship. We have a mutual love of the bush, and along with that, perhaps, a certain dread of it. If we have not shared discomforts and joys shoulder to shoulder, we have shared some of them, nevertheless, though widely separated, I trust that we will share them further occasionally in the future.[4]

Flynn's reference to a love of the bush working hand in hand with a 'certain dread of it' is a theme that recurs in much of his writing, and his desire to eliminate this dread underscores a great deal of his later efforts on behalf of the Inlanders. By modern standards, the text of *The Bushman's Companion* may seem rather quaint, but there can be no doubt that it was heartfelt. For example, in the part entitled 'A Ramble Among Ideals', his homespun homilies include 'The Man Who Tries Again', 'The Man Who Aims High', 'The Man Who Plods Ever Forward', and sweetly, 'The Man Who Maintains in Himself What He Demands in Woman'.[5]

In the section on first aid, the instructions were carefully phrased. An intuitive teacher, Flynn realised the wisdom of introducing a new concept by invoking one already understood. 'Common sense will not altogether fail when a breakdown occurs. The man who can splint up the shaft of a dray should surely be able to splint up a broken leg! He will use different splints and bandages, and will pad everything in the most careful way; but the main principle is really similar.'[6]

The Bushman's Companion was free of charge although its users were invited to donate a trifle to its production if they wished. It was a huge success and may well have brought home to Flynn the importance of the written word in reaching out to people. Later, in *The Inlander* magazine, to which he was chief contributor and editor, he used this practice to great effect.

Other plans were also being hatched. Flynn decided that a Mailbag League should be instigated to encourage people in the populated areas to send letters and news to those in the bush. In this way it was hoped to break down the feeling of isolation which was the bushman's constant companion. In this endeavour Flynn enlisted the help of a group of women, including his sister Rosetta, who was often to be involved, sometimes unwillingly, in Flynn's many projects. Flynn hoped that the scheme would go beyond women writing to women and asks in *The Bushman's Companion*, 'Are there no isolated men in the back of beyond who would like to correspond with other fellows down South?'[7] Flynn's desire to give the bush a voice began here and culminated in the creation of a radio network throughout the Inland.

Thus, Flynn's consciousness of how he might serve the people of the Inland began to grow. Unwittingly, he was sowing the seeds for a much more ambitious program from which the people of the outback would reap a rich harvest. But for the moment, there were his final examinations at Ormond to complete. Having scraped through, he was finally ordained into the Presbyterian Church on 24 January 1911. He was thirty-one years old. In February the Rev. John Flynn arrived at Beltana, in northern South Australia, to undertake missionary work at the Smith of Dunesk mission. He took over the job from the Rev. E Baldwin who had earlier intimated to Flynn that he had earmarked the young missionary as his successor. It was to be a two-year posting. Flynn was to be based at a manse in Beltana and from there to minister to a large region stretching into the remote areas of the state.

This was a region that was sparsely populated, one person per every 21 square kilometres. By dint of their small numbers, pioneers in the small settlements and workers on the pastoral stations lacked the clout to force the interest of governments or indeed of most citizens in the more populous areas. The church, too, had little involvement and vast areas of the outback were almost entirely untended by any of the religious denominations.

So the Smith of Dunesk mission was somewhat of a rarity in what it was attempting to do. It had come about, not through the instigation of any local church group, but because of the largesse of a Scottish woman, Mrs Henrietta Smith of Dunesk Manor, near Edinburgh. The mission, established in 1893, was named in her honour after she bequeathed means to the Free Church of Scotland for the benefit of the colony of South Australia.

From Beltana, Flynn travelled in the mission's battered old two-horse buggy weighed down with swag, waterbag, tuckerbox, cooking implements, feed for the horses, camera, books and magazines for the settlers starved for reading material, and a supply of *The Bushman's Companion*. He ventured as far north as Oodnadatta and to the east to the Queensland border, visiting homesteads and small settlements, and observing first hand the rigours of the bushman's life. The variety of topography – gibber plains, sandhills, grasslands, and creeks that were impassable when rain fell – made travel by horsedrawn vehicle difficult. Motor transport, rarely used, fared no better.

A most pressing problem was that of communication. Mail arrived infrequently, visitors were few. The vagaries of the mail delivery were a concern to women relying on the post for medical supplies for their family. One woman describes her experience in a letter dated 1 March 1913: 'I have a parcel of medicines somewhere along the road between here and Oodnadatta, which I ordered on 16 December 1912. These were for myself and child, who was then about three weeks old. The latest advice I have about these medicines is that they will not be here for three weeks yet.'[8]

The Overland Telegraph Line stretching from Darwin to Adelaide was the lifeline by which settlers could keep in touch with the outside world and summon help when it was needed. Even this, though, was of limited value, since the telegraph repeating stations were positioned at 160-kilometre intervals along the line with the journey to them long and arduous over roads that were mere tracks, carved out by the passage of whatever camel train, bullock wagon or buggy had gone before. And beneath the trees and beside the dry creek beds and rough tracks were solitary bush graves – unmarked or bearing a simple wooden cross – testament to the lonely deaths of pioneers starved of medical assistance.

The railway from Adelaide was a boon but it stopped at Oodnadatta. If a sick or injured person needed to be transported to a station along the line, often a great distance, the effect on the patient of the journey in a jolting conveyance could be at best painful, at worst fatal. The following account illustrates the point:

> As regards the report you ask me to send you about our little child's death, I hardly know how to start it, but she took very suddenly ill on Monday 13 December, at half past three in the afternoon, and we left our home on Tuesday after dinner for our journey of 59 to 60 miles for Hergott. We stayed at _____ on Tuesday night, as the dear little child seemed much better. But at 12 o'clock she took a turn for the worse, so we left at half past 12 in the night for Hergott Springs; but being so dark and dry we lost the road – and delayed our journey a few hours. At last we found the road, and after passing the netting fence we had the misfortune to have an accident, being thrown from the trap into a

watercourse, but as nothing serious happened, we continued our journey, but just got within sight of the railway in time to see the South train leave for Quorn. As no other train was leaving for the South we had to wait with our sick child until a special sheep train on Thursday 16th, and it being six hours late, we arrived in Hawker (150 miles south) six hours late, and the poor little child died one and a half hours before Hawker was reached. I must also say if a doctor had been at Hergott we would have had the dear little bright and happy girl until this day, but, as in all other sickness you have to go so far for a doctor, Hawker being the nearest, I think it time that the Government put some one in charge at Hergott. Our little Mary was just twelve months old, convulsions caused her death, and how I miss her no one knows.[9]

This was the type of situation which Flynn observed and about which he longed to take remedial action. He began to dream about a network of cottage hospitals, scattered throughout the hinterland, which would provide nursing care to those within their radius, and compensate in part for the absence of doctors. A start had been made at Oodnadatta in the appointment of a nursing sister, Sister Alice Main, by an early Smith of Dunesk missionary. Without a proper building in which to minister to the sick, Sister Main cared for patients in their homes. She was succeeded by a nurse-deaconess, Sister Latto Bett. When Flynn arrived at Dunesk, the inadequacy of the nursing arrangements had been acknowledged and plans were under way to build a medical hostel in Oodnadatta. Two hundred and fourteen pounds had been raised towards this endeavour. Although the amount was not sufficient to complete the job, Flynn, in his indomitable fashion, forged ahead regardless. Plans were drawn up for an appropriate building and, when an anonymous donation of £400 was received, work began in earnest. Throughout his life of service, Flynn held the belief that providence would supply whatever funds were needed for the execution of his plans. Perhaps this conviction stemmed from the mysterious appearance of the £400!

2

The Kirk at Work

. . . .

As well as carrying out his duties at Beltana, Flynn supervised the building project at Oodnadatta, and watched with satisfaction as the small, galvanised iron hospital took shape. It was opened in December 1911 as the temperature soared to 106 degrees and torrential rain beat down a benediction. The Rev. Robert Mitchell, the very first Smith of Dunesk missionary, was the guest of honour and explained to the gathering what might be expected of Sister Bett: 'Nurse Bett is sister-in-charge of the Hostel. Here she will do her best for all who seek her services as a duly qualified nurse. She is also a deaconess of the Presbyterian Church, and will exercise her high office in the interests of all, without preference for nationality or creed. Her business is not to tamper with the beliefs of patients, but to surround them with a womanly Christian influence.'[1] By all accounts, Nurse Bett and those who succeeded her took this instruction to heart and carried out their work with dedication and distinction.

Two years later Flynn gives a fascinating description of the cottage hospital which became a prototype for those that followed:

> There is a house 35 × 33 feet, with ward, dispensary, bathroom,
> hall, sitting room, bedroom, kitchen, scullery, 10 foot wide

verandah all round, washhouse, isolation tent, lawn – yes, a living, live, thirsty lawn. Fortunately Oodnadatta has a fine bore near by, and water is laid on all over the township. The water contains some soda and other minerals, but most people can take tea made from it, and most plant life flourishes fairly well by its aid – some shrubs and pot plants; furnishings and hangings in all rooms; and dust-storms occasionally; but no maid, not even a permanent lubra. To save labour the Nurse 'has meals out', and only invalid food is prepared on the premises as a rule.[2]

In addition to caring for the sick, the nurse's duties were to distribute parcels of books, teach bible lessons to the children each morning, conduct services on Sunday and provide hospitality for any wayfarer who dropped by keen to enjoy this little oasis of sociability.

A hospital like this was an example of the practical Christianity which Flynn had been practising since the beginning of his home mission career. In his travels he had become acutely conscious of the lengths to which men would go to reach medical aid. Stories abounded of outback men carrying a sick or injured mate over hundreds of kilometres of inhospitable country just to reach someone with even a rudimentary knowledge of first aid. He doubted that such an effort would be made to visit a church. However, if the two concepts could be married, such that the church was seen to provide medical care and solicitude, then the bushman's attention to spiritual concerns might follow consequentially. The average bushman was not a verbose man. Isolation, the lack of community life and the absence of recreational activities meant that social skills were not honed – and his trust was not easily won. Action rather than words would be required to win his notice.

The loneliness of the outback and the fear of what might happen to loved ones with almost no access to medical help was a mitigating factor against people taking on the Inland as a place to live and rear families. The ratio of men to women was overwhelmingly in favour of the former whose mantra was that the bush was 'no place for a woman'. In *We of the Never-Never*, the author, Mrs Aeneas Gunn, records her husband as saying, 'The average bushman will face fire and flood, hunger and even death itself, to help the frail or weak ones who come into his life; although he'll strive to the utmost to keep the Unknown Woman out of his environments, particularly when those environments are a hundred miles from anywhere.'[3] This was borne out by the pastoralists' tendency to favour the employment of single men, or in advertising for a married couple, to add the stipulation 'No encumbrances'. However, argued Flynn, if Australians were to consider themselves custodians of this vast continent, then they had a duty to settle it comprehensively. Flynn set great store by the capacity of women and children to have a civilising effect simply by being present. 'It is a rare thing for a bushman to be rude to a woman – even when he is drunk – and a rarer to hear him using bad language in her presence,' wrote an experienced bush traveller.[4] Nonetheless, men were reluctant to bring women into the outback and women were reluctant to raise children in such a harsh environment. If nursing care were more readily available, Flynn thought this situation could be addressed. Flynn's sensitivity to the vulnerability of women in the outback may have resulted from the loss of his own mother, who died in childbirth in 1883 when he was an infant. He held the view that with families came a feeling of permanence and stability which would encourage the growth of communities. Such a measure would in turn help populate the interior. And this, Flynn believed, was Australia's economic and moral obligation.

Even before he went to Beltana, Flynn had been amassing material about the outback, much of which had emanated from his request to readers of *The Bushman's Companion* to send along information, suggestions, and particulars of their needs. He continued this process after his arrival. Also of crucial importance to the development of his thinking had been a letter from a Mrs Jessie Litchfield of Port Darwin, received by the editor of *The Messenger*, the journal of the

Presbyterian Church of Victoria, and handed on to Flynn.[5] In it was sketched a vivid and very raw (for its day) picture of conditions in the far north and the licentious behaviour of its inhabitants. She urged the church to send a missionary to the Northern Territory to give moral and spiritual guidance. This plea had stayed in Flynn's mind. While ministering to Central Australia, Flynn hoped to somehow draw the Northern Territory within his sphere of influence. He was keen to make a report of the outback to raise awareness of the needs of the Inlanders. Friends at home worked behind the scenes, promoting the idea and raising funds for its execution.

In April 1912 a joint conference of the Victorian Home Mission Committee and the Australian Board of Missions took up the challenge to survey conditions in the Northern Territory. Flynn was commissioned for the job and was to report to the next Federal Assembly of the Presbyterian Church. He viewed the assignment with delight and not a little trepidation.

He set sail for Darwin and for seven weeks branched out from this base to make trips south to Katherine River, west to the settlement on Daly River, east among the small mining camps out of Pine Creek, north to Bathurst Island, and again round from Darwin by sea to Adelaide River. He travelled by train, buckboard, lugger and motorboat.

His report was called *Northern Territory and Central Australia: A Call to the Church*. It was an original and comprehensive work, painting a picture of the working and living conditions he had observed, the potential for the development of pastoral and mining industries, and the pressing need for an expanded railway and communication system if the twin problems of isolation and distance were to be overcome. With no rail link between the south and the far north, Flynn felt that Darwin had virtually been cut loose from the rest of Australia. Flynn asserted, 'I believe there are great things in store for the Northern Territory as a whole, but citizens of Australia must be prepared to purchase the future.'[6] He saw three main problems for the Territory –

rainfall (high on the coast, meagre in the interior), absence of markets, and scarcity of labour. While the church could do little about these issues, it could help in more humanitarian ways. First, he recommended that two travelling ministers be appointed, one to work out of Pine Creek, south of Darwin, and the other out of Oodnadatta. They would patrol the hinterland of Australia in the same way as Flynn and his predecessors had done in a more limited way at Smith of Dunesk. Second, he wanted to build on the goodwill that the Presbyterian Church had already achieved via the work of the deaconess-nurse in Oodnadatta by finding a person willing to carry out similar work in Alice Springs. Third, he wanted the church to be national in its approach to the welfare of the people of the outback and for the scope of the work not to be limited by state borders. And finally, he recommended that a stock of books be made available to the Inlanders, a 'road' library, chosen to appeal to all reading tastes, with a direction on each volume that it be passed on when read.

Not content with the excursion he had just made, he proposed a further journey to examine areas he had not yet visited – an ambitious scope – from Oodnadatta via Alice Springs to Pine Creek (near Darwin); across to Burketown (on the Gulf of Carpentaria); southward via Camooweal, Cloncurry, Birdsville (in Queensland); to Innamincka (near the Queensland border); and Broken Hill (in New South Wales). He concluded the report by warning, 'Difficulties of a serious nature will arise in shoals in every fertile mind. To each one a reply can only be made in words already familiar, "Do not pray for tasks equal to your powers; pray for powers equal to your tasks".'[7]

Flynn's recommendations were well received and the General Assembly constituted the Northern Territory with extensive portions of adjacent states a special sphere for Christian work. The task was a mammoth one. The area under consideration covered half the Australian continent and, to increase the unwieldiness, inhabitants were not in large groups but clustered in twos and tens and twenties throughout the region. Undaunted, the Assembly appointed Flynn as head of the organisation that would undertake this work. It was later named the Australian Inland Mission (AIM) – the 'bush department' of the Presbyterian Church. Flynn was to hold the position of super-intendent for the next thirty-nine years. Out of this role and through his tireless pursuit of a better deal for bush people would come the moniker 'Flynn of the Inland'.

The Assembly decided that in order to realise their ambitions, a considerable sum of money would be needed. A Bush Brigade was planned to raise money for Flynn's proposals with the hope that 5000 members of the church could be persuaded to pledge one pound per year. A Bush Committee was formed to control the project.

Flynn was eager to return to the Inland but there were other more pressing tasks. He was needed to work on the organisational details of the AIM, to promote its existence to a wider audience than the church, and to encourage donations for the project's implementation. And a missionary had to be found to take over the work at Smith of Dunesk in Flynn's absence.

Among the group that gathered to witness the public launching of the AIM was a young lay preacher, Robert Bruce Plowman, who listened intently to the words of Flynn and the other outback advo-cates. Inspired by what he heard, he was keen to sign up. Despite the initial intention to use only ordained ministers, the Home Mission Board were impressed by Plowman's youth, vigour and enthusiasm, and gave him the job. In any case, regular ministers were not rushing to volunteer, perhaps being chary of such a difficult assignment when there were comfortable suburban parishes on offer.

Plowman arrived at Beltana in November 1912 and in the follow-ing twelve months journeyed by horse and buggy to the furthest reaches of the Smith of Dunesk boundaries and beyond. In late 1913 he transferred to the AIM and was encouraged by Flynn to press on beyond Oodnadatta and into the Northern Territory. This was camel country. Camels can be unruly animals – 'brutes' as Plowman frequently described them – but he learned to drive his team along in a masterly fashion, even developing a certain admiration for the camels' recalcitrance. His passage was not an easy one. He had to find his way over tracks that were almost non-existent and discover the whereabouts of the waterholes that spelt the difference between life and death – and there was the possibility of attacks from hostile Aboriginal groups. As a safeguard, and unusually for a churchman, Plowman carried a revolver. In this and in his behaviour and appearance generally, he did not fit the usual mental picture of a travelling missionary. He took a leaf out of Flynn's book and always offered practical help before spiritual help, rolling up his sleeves and good-naturedly working alongside the men when the opportunity arose. 'The preacher must prove that he was a man first of all, capable of standing on his own feet, and with a good sense of humour. This earned him the right to speak in due season'.[8] The tasks he was called upon to perform were many. He helped with mustering, yarding, shoeing, branding and well-sinking, and carried news, messages and letters from one location to another. His usefulness also went indoors, where he nursed the sick as best he could, gave lessons and told bible stories to the station children, and mended household items. This particular talent brought him more than he had bargained for when visiting a station in the MacDonnell Ranges. He successfully mended the gramophone and within minutes 'a handleless flour scoop, a tin kettle with a detached spout, several tin dishes with holes in them – in fact about everything on the station that had come unstuck or had sprung a leak, had been assembled and planted down in front of the astounded mechanic'.[9]

Plowman rejoiced in religious expression in whatever form he found it. On his first visit to Birdsville in Queensland he noted: 'At the service that night the townspeople attended without respect of denominational difference … On our expressing pleasure at such a happy state of religious concord, the people told us that they have so few services that they all gladly attend whatever services are held.'[10]

When Plowman left the field after five years, he used the details of his experiences as the basis for a trilogy of books which gave readers, sometimes for the first time, a glimpse of the harsh conditions of the outback and the exceptional qualities of the outback people.

Plowman was a test case for the AIM. If he was able to demonstrate the value of ministering to the Inlanders, no matter how few their numbers or how remote their habitats, then support for patrolling padres would be strengthened. Positive feedback from the field indicated that he had done just that. Plowman was succeeded by the Rev. Kingsley 'Skipper' Partridge who was to devote many years of his life to patrolling the same area with a similar attention to presenting himself as the sort of bushman to whom outback people could relate.

While Plowman was thus successfully engaged, the new superintendent of the AIM was continuing his propaganda and fundraising activities on the coast. He travelled extensively from Adelaide to Townsville, by road, rail and sea, seeking publicity and mustering support. He lectured tirelessly, using his maps and lantern slides as visual aids to illustrate his outback anecdotes. Progress was slow, so it was fortunate that Flynn was a patient man.

Early in 1913, Flynn put his fundraising duties on hold and set out for his long-awaited tour of the north of Central Australia. Regrettably there was insufficient time for the more ambitious itinerary that he had signalled in his 1912 report to the General Assembly. However, in order to further champion the Inlanders' cause, he felt an obligation, and desire, to see more of their living conditions. Although he was well travelled, there were still large slabs of the outback which Flynn had not examined at first hand. This was to be his first trip beyond Oodnadatta to the fledgling settlement of Alice Springs, in the very heart of the continent.

In the initial stage he travelled by coach and then joined Texas, an outback mailman, on a camel trek. Flynn was captivated by what he saw – both the beauty *and* the terror. His descriptions are full and arresting, and demonstrate his rather wry sense of humour. For example, in his account of the area around Oodnadatta, he gives this description:

> At Oodnadatta one looks every way over 'gibber' plains. In one direction a belt of stunted timber marks the Neale River, which is true Australian in that it runs only when in the humour. In places flat-topped and very low hills are observed. They look as if decaying yet, and so they are. The gibbers are smooth water-worn stones, and are found for most part on the surface only. When one gets beyond the working radius of township goats, saltbush may be seen, and after rain sweet picking of grass is along all the depressions. But rain is not regular. It comes just often enough to keep up an average of four inches a year, and is some-times too busy elsewhere to come at all for a year at a time.[11]

The trip culminated in Alice Springs where Flynn found much to appeal, challenging the reader to find it otherwise. 'Alice Springs prepares one for something pleasant, and pleasant that part of the world is to an Inlander. Those folk who expect babbling brooks at springs, murmuring streams at rivers, snow-clad heights in ranges, and English meadows in Australia, will never altogether approve of Alice Springs and MacDonnell Ranges. Well they can stay away'.[12] Thus began Flynn's love affair with Alice Springs. It was here that the most ambitious of the AIM hospitals would be built and here where John Flynn's ashes would ultimately be laid to rest.

Flynn was fulsome in his praise of the water quality in the township wells and the condition of the soil which allowed for the cultivation of fruit and vegetables for those inclined to put in the work. He was entranced by the bold outline of the MacDonnell Ranges which formed the background of the township. And he was moved afresh by the character of the bushman and the stoic way in which he handled deprivation. 'When rain keeps away so persistently the people try to look cheerful, and succeed. When rain comes they look cheerful without trying. It is bad form to whine, and your form must be of a thorough quality to be good enough for the bush.'[13]

Flynn thought that Australians would be remiss in their duty if they did not care for these exceptional people. 'Our special interest is in the men and women and children who live in those lonely spaces. We are not throwing our sympathy at them, for they live on the whole very happily, and are perhaps more cheerful than we. All honour to them! But what about *our* honour?'[14] That the 'honour' of Flynn and his collaborators was upheld in ensuing years was confirmed beyond doubt by their unflagging dedication to the Inlanders' cause.

3

A Voice for the Outback

. . . .

Flynn decided that a vehicle was needed by which the outback could tell its own story to the wider public and press its case for greater consideration. On his return from Alice Springs, he proposed to the Home Mission Board a quarterly bush magazine to be called *The Inlander*. His advocacy was successful and the magazine made its first appearance in November 1913. It appeared regularly until 1918 and then sporadically until 1929, as Flynn's focus was diverted elsewhere. On its title page it claimed, 'Like other bush travellers, *The Inlander* appears when best it can'.

The Inlander was to become a manifesto of Flynn's vision for the outback. It was peppered with discourses on agriculture, politics and economics, and descriptions of flora, fauna and family life where it existed. It also contained maps (Flynn became a quite competent cartographer), tables of rainfalls, population densities and temperature patterns, and even pages of interest to children. The details came from what Flynn learned and observed during his exhaustive travelling and from material supplied by others. As an educational tool it was of great importance as very little real information about the outback had previously been available.

The lively descriptions of the Inlanders and their mode of living were designed to capture the hearts and minds of city readers and gently guide them into identifying more fully with the struggles of their country counterparts. The strategy seemed to work as the magazine made frequent references to donations big and small from a disparate group of readers, including those who had nothing to gain personally from such largesse. The evocative reportage of far-flung regions and interesting choice of words, Darwin for instance was 'Australia's front door', encouraged readers to conceptualise these places. If readers could not call there in person, they could visit in their imagination.

Flynn was an expert photographer and shared the pictorial records of what he saw with his readers. These photos are a fascinating chronicle of the outback. They show the starkness of the townships – often ramshackle groups of buildings perched in the middle of nowhere – and the sparseness of the countryside. His writing demonstrated an intense interest in what made outback people tick and a keen observance of their habits and behaviour. He had a touching concern for their comfort and living arrangements, seeming to take great pleasure in finding a well-designed house, or a garden coaxed into bloom in the most severe temperatures by the lady of the house. His compassion is evident in a photo of a rudimentary dwelling with a couple at the door and a line of washing in the foreground. The description on the facing page reads: 'Real, all too real, is the mud which lies thick in the primitive backyard, and invades the kitchen-vestibule-scullery-storeroom-dining-reception room all day long in spite of attempts to keep it back. Real, also, are those heavy garments which regularly come along for cleansing, and provide hard toil to save the woman from brooding overmuch about her troubles.'[1]

As a publicist Flynn was a natural. The exposure which the stories in The Inlander received in various periodicals – both church and secular – was designed to make going to the Inland heroic at the outset – and later entirely familiar by dint of Flynn's constant descriptions of

the look and daily doings in these isolated regions. He intended this
propaganda to work on the minds of both adults and children. There
are frequent stories of children donating their small allowances to the
cause or raising money in innovative ways. This account is illustrative:
'The Sunday School at Coonamble, NSW, wants to have a camel. The
young people are modest, however, for if they can merely own him,
and have his photo to admire, they will then allow an AIM missionary
to ride him. So far they have bought one leg at £3/11/-, and are
eager to get the other three legs and all the rest – for you cannot take
delivery in instalments.'[2]

The magazine praised the efforts of the bush men and women and
also gave space to stories illustrating the unique quality of children
reared in the outback. An example was that of a family of young
children living in the goldfields of Western Australia who discovered
their mother dead from heat apoplexy. With the father away prospecting, the eldest child, Vincent, made the decision to fetch help.

> He decided to go to his uncle at the Five Mile, taking the
> younger children with him. He first fed the poultry, gave them
> water, turned the windmill off, gave each of the children a piece
> of bread and butter and a drink of water, taking a big drink
> himself to see him through the journey. He then filled the water
> bag and got a bottle for the baby to drink from, put the baby into
> a go-cart, which he pushed, and, for fear it would perish if left
> behind, took a young puppy with them. Between 1.30 and 2 pm
> the sad little procession started out for the Empress mine, over
> five miles away, bare-footed, and through sand, with the
> thermometer registering 110 degrees in the shade. This little
> band consisted of Vincent, aged 10 years, Robert aged 8, Isabel
> aged 5, Arthur aged 3, and the baby aged 7 months. The puppy
> was the first to knock up and had to be carried; then Arthur,
> whose feet were badly blistered, had to be taken up. Vincent, with
> his young brother on his back, and pushing the go-cart through

the sand, became greatly distressed, but pushed manfully on. With the extreme heat the baby required every attention and a sip of water every few hundred yards. Vincent's great anxiety was that the water bag would give out before they reached the Five Mile, but he brought his little expedition safely through, and they arrived at about 5 pm, when he reported the sad news and obtained assistance.[3]

Reading such stories, it would be hard to argue against the need for greater support for the bush. *The Inlander* magazine logged every painstaking step in Flynn's plans to create a 'mantle of safety' over the Inland. And its readers came along for the ride. The first volumes established the credentials of the outback and the people who lived there. Successive volumes described the network of the AIM cottage hospitals that gradually appeared throughout the interior, applauded the work of the expanding band of nursing sisters and patrol padres, and ultimately followed the difficult task of taking the network of care from the ground into the air when the aerial medical service took flight. Throughout every volume was a sense of Flynn's strengthening conviction that only the best was good enough for the bush and that a visionary approach was needed to achieve it.

The highlight of 1914 for Flynn was a four-month visit to the far north-west of Western Australia. Here, Flynn had two more travelling padres working under his jurisdiction, in addition to Plowman in Central Australia, and he was keen to see them in action. Jim Stevens was based at Port Hedland in the Pilbara, patrolling his area with some originality in a buggy drawn by two camels, and Frank Brady was in Broome, travelling around his parish in a more orthodox horsedrawn buggy.

Flynn travelled by mailboat from Fremantle to Broome, the centre of a thriving pearling industry. As usual, Flynn found much there to stimulate his fertile mind and devoted space in *The Inlander* to sharing the details of the pearlers and their equipment and the perils that they confronted, every bit as dangerous, Flynn concluded, as those that beset the miners in their industry. Brady patrolled the vast Kimberley area and conducted church services for the many itinerant pearlers in Broome. His supply of books and magazines was also a comfort to the men who ruefully reported that in the absence of any other reading matter they had taken to reading the labels of jam jars – and then reading them again.

From Broome, Flynn sailed back down the coast to Port Hedland where he found Padre Stevens making lengthy treks to visit his constituents, including one notable trip of 1600 kilometres. Stevens reports, 'This trip took me on to the edge of the desert, beyond the last fence, and to the farthest-out settlers. One brave-hearted woman had lived out on the desert for four years, and had only seen one other white woman during that time, and that when she had visited a neighbouring station to record her vote.'[4] Here again was evidence of the effort required to carry out the most commonplace activity, underscored by the insidious problems of isolation and distance. According to Flynn, it was distance that was killing the Inland.

From Port Hedland, Flynn arrived in Kalgoorlie to inspect the construction camps on the western end of the transcontinental railway that was to link Port Augusta with Kalgoorlie. This nation-building endeavour had first been mooted many years before, surveys had begun in 1909, and the difficult construction started to inch its way across the desert in 1912. An ecumenical mission had been established to cater to the needs of the railway workers and Flynn was impressed with the work it did in providing activities for the men at the end of a day of difficult and back-breaking work. Each week as the railway line progressed, the camp would be shifted further along the track and the recreation tent, which offered cards, draughts, gramophone, reading matter and writing materials, would move with it. These pursuits, along with church services on Sunday, reinforced the idea among the men that an interest was being taken in their social and spiritual welfare. It was practical Christianity at work.

By the time Flynn reported to the General Assembly later that year, Australia was at war. Flynn was acutely conscious of the difficulties of asking the public, seized with patriotic fervour, to direct attention and funds to those on the home front when men were embarking to fight on battlefields abroad. He knew also that the war effort would swallow up chaplains and nurses to serve overseas who might otherwise have considered joining the ranks of the AIM. And there would be the defection of those already in the field. Jim Stevens left his post at Port Hedland to enlist, vowing to return when the conflict was over, but was killed conducting a field burial in France in 1918. Yet Flynn was aware that when the war ended, many who had signed up would re-settle in the outback, where their needs would be as pressing as ever.

Flynn's message was that people served their country in various capacities and that it was not only war that separated families. In the previous year he had made that point eloquently.

> One man may serve his country seeing that our cables,
> transferred to the wire at Darwin, are still safe when they reach
> the Centre – and send his son away 1,000 miles to Adelaide to
> attend school, while his wife works out her calculations of the
> heart to decide whether she will follow her little boy or stand by
> her husband. Another man may serve his country by supervising
> the police of 250,000 miles of Our Country – and send his five
> children away from *their* rightful protector and chum all the way
> to Sydney again, and exile their mother with them. Another man
> may serve his country growing beef for the ever hungry people
> of the city – and send his children away, 1,000 miles away, after
> the beef.[5]

This was the tenor of his thinking, and in submitting his report, Flynn did not shrink from outlining the various problems the AIM was encountering – difficulty with recruitment, lack of financial support, thousands of people scattered throughout the outback, still lacking spiritual and medical support, and the problem of the immense areas that had to be serviced. He was fond of saying that within the AIM's enormous sphere could be placed the British Isles, France, Germany, Austria-Hungary, Luxembourg, Belgium, Holland, Denmark, Norway, Sweden, Switzerland, Italy, Spain, Portugal, Albania, Yugoslavia, Montenegro, Serbia, Romania, Bulgaria, Greece, Turkey and Italy and then 'you would have to stow in Monaco and a quarter of Russia by way of filling up the cracks'.[6] It was a graphic way to make the point.

Nonetheless, he saw reason for hope in the five excellent workers who had already been brought under the AIM's umbrella – layman (Robert) Bruce Plowman patrolling in Central Australia, Sister Latto Bett at the hostel in Oodnadatta, and three ministers. (Brady and Stevens had been joined by the Rev. JC Gibson who had signed up for Pine Creek, two years after Flynn had indicated this need in his 1912 report.) And *The Inlander* continued to do successful work in engaging the public's interest. Flynn went on to boldly propose an increase in the number of patrol padres and nursing sisters and an expansion in building work. And he confidently asserted that it would all be financed by 'a revolution in Home Mission thinking, feeling and giving'. The Assembly reeled at his audacity – and reappointed him superintendent for another two years.

During the war years, progress was slow but steady as Flynn fought tirelessly for a share of public sympathy for his beloved Inlanders. Deluged with paperwork, he organised volunteer Office Teams to work in the city offices helping with correspondence and accounts and the organisation of fundraising activities. The Office Teams also looked after the job of packing and distributing the avalanche of books which arrived constantly from supporters and which were destined for readers in the outback. A photo in *The Inlander* shows the output – an enormous pile of brown paper packages of all shapes and sizes ready for despatch.

Dissatisfied with the disproportionate number of patrol padres to nursing sisters, Flynn became increasingly preoccupied with developing a network of cottage hospitals, each one to be strategically placed to service a radius of 400 or 500 kilometres. He envisaged these bases as the hubs of many wheels of medical attention. They were difficult to get under way unless concerned people agitated for them in their own locality. And governments were uninterested in building uneconomic hospitals in sparsely populated areas. '[So Flynn] determined that the AIM should do the pioneering work for them. But with this difference: the AIM hostel (or nursing home) would be more than a medical institution; it would be a social, cultural and religious centre as well.'[7] To this end in 1915 a hostel was established in a rented building at Port Hedland in north-west Western Australia, with Flynn undertaking to find a suitable nurse to run it.

The establishment of the next two cottage hospitals was prompted by local crises. Padre Gibson, patrolling his parish from Pine Creek in the Northern Territory, discovered an unusual lull in the activity of the tin fields of Maranboy. He learned that an outbreak of fever had cut a swath through the miners and several had died. Gibson suggested engaging an AIM sister so that nursing care would be available should such an epidemic recur. The miners were to help raise the funds for a building. The hat was passed around and the AIM's third cottage hospital was under way with Sister Hepburn and a companion May Gillespie in charge. Subsequently there was another outbreak of fever during which nineteen in-patients and numerous outpatients were treated. This time there were no fatalities.

Miss Gillespie described conditions at the Maranboy hospital, illustrating how adept she and her companion were at looking on the positive side of their rather difficult existence:

> We have water laid on and electric light; at the battery manager's
> house they have electric fans, ice machines and gramophones, so
> we are not quite out of civilisation, though we are 250 miles from

Darwin, and 50 miles from the nearest railway. All the stores are carried out by teams, either horse or donkey. The donkey team is quite picturesque – 26 donkeys, three abreast, and all with names! We have to get in a supply of stores to last over the wet season, i.e., four of five months, as the roads get too bad for the teamsters. We have a mail coach once a week to and from Katherine, but are only getting a Southern mail every four or five weeks at present.[8]

Testament to the excellent work of the two women was a letter received at the end of their posting from the residents of the township:

To Nurse Hepburn and Miss Gillespie,

We, the residents of Marranboy, who have been the recipients of your continual courtesy and consideration, desire on the eve of your departure to present you with a tangible form of our appreciation, and hand you herewith the sum of seventy pounds five shillings contributed with a whole-hearted unanimity by the Marranboy Tinfield.

Since your advent the conditions socially and otherwise have shown an unmistakable improvement, and your professional services have this year averted a catastrophe.

You leave this way-back centre with the good wishes of every resident, not only locally, but in the surrounding district.

Your stay has made for good, and in regretting your departure we sincerely wish you both God-speed.[9]

Clearly the townsfolk were appreciative of the difficult work of the nursing sister. The nurses were generally cheerful in their reports but they faced pressures that could at times be debilitating. They had to contend with the privation of living far from their personal and professional support groups, while assuming responsibility for the sick and injured, with no doctor on hand to provide medical backup.

Difficult decisions often had to be made between staying at the hospital to receive patients or leaving on an arduous trek to care for a critical patient some distance away. And after embarking on such a mercy mission there might be the heartbreak of arriving too late to save a life. Aware of this burden, Flynn decided that all cottage hospitals should have two women in attendance, either two nurses or a nurse and a companion. Even if the companion were not trained in hospital work, they would at least provide company and moral support. Later the stipulation became for two trained nurses.

4

The Tyranny of Distance

. . . .

The establishment of a fourth hostel at Halls Creek in Western Australia was the result of an incident in 1917 which focused minds once more on the inadequacy of medical facilities in the outback. A young stockman named Jimmy Darcy had fallen heavily from his horse and was badly injured. His mates made the decision to transport him by buggy to the postmaster at Halls Creek, Fred Tuckett, the only person within a 400-kilometre radius with any knowledge of first aid. It took many hours before Darcy's helpmates were ready to set out and another twelve hours before the telegraph office was reached – an excruciatingly painful journey for the hapless Darcy. Tuckett examined Darcy as best he could and sought help by telegraph from Wyndham and Derby – to no avail. In desperation Tuckett decided to telegraph Dr John Holland in Perth from whom he had received first aid instruction some years before. Tuckett no doubt began to regret his reputation as a bush doctor for Dr Holland diagnosed a ruptured bladder and insisted that Tuckett operate. Tuckett protested that he had no surgical equipment but the reply tapped back over a distance of 3200 kilometres was unequivocal – operate or the young man will die. Having given Darcy morphia to ease the pain, and using a sharpened penknife as an instrument, the amateur surgeon carried out the operation, following instructions relayed back and forth down the telegraph wire by morse code. The procedure was successful but Darcy remained in a critical condition. Dr Holland, whose interest had been piqued by the case, decided to take on Darcy's post-operative care himself. His mercy mission by boat, car and horse took twelve days. Finally Holland arrived at Halls Creek and asked, 'How is the patient?' Came Tuckett's sorrowful reply, 'He died yesterday morning'.

Extraordinarily, the operation had been successful but Darcy had died from complications caused by undiagnosed malaria. Today his gravestone stands in the cemetery in Halls Creek and reads simply: 'Sacred to the memory of James Darcy, who died at Halls Creek 22 August 1917, aged 29 years. RIP'. Dr B Cohen, writing in *The Medical Journal of Australia* at the time of Dr Holland's death, estimated the total cost of the wires sent back and forth was £600; the first wire had totalled 279 words.[1] When Dr Holland arrived back in Perth he was met by John Flynn who was making one of his periodic visits to Perth. Jean Lang, writing in *Early Days*, the journal of the Royal Western Australian Historical Society, recorded Holland's comment to Flynn on being asked about his mercy mission: 'Everywhere I went, the men asked me to return, but next time I'll fly'.[2] No doubt this comment was tucked away in Flynn's mind and may have played a part in his later advocacy for flying doctors.

Again the problem of distance was seen as the root cause of this tragic and unnecessary death and focused attention on the need for more readily available medical assistance. Why, asked Flynn, should the pioneers always have to pay for the nation's development – with courage, with toil, with the sacrifice of everyday comforts, with life they should never have to give? The incident was widely reported and tugged at the heartstrings of everyone who heard of it. In the Halls Creek district, Tuckett and others agitated for a cottage hospital and in the following year a public meeting decided that one should be established. It was housed in the Halls Creek Miners' Institute Hall and again Flynn arranged for the staffing. Throughout his time at

Halls Creek, Fred Tuckett was understandably one of the hospital's staunchest supporters.

The demands of war, in terms of medical, material and human resources curbed Flynn's ambitions, but also drew attention to burgeoning aviation activity and its possibilities for peace work – and Flynn, never slow to seize the initiative, began to press the advantage. Flynn's personal battle, fought on the home front, was to demonstrate how aeroplanes might be used in the service of the Inland. He imagined flying doctors working from a central base, not unlike the nursing sisters, and swooping down to administer to the sick, to dispense advice and medication, and to carry off the serious cases to the closest hospital.

Seminal was a letter received by Flynn from a Lieutenant Clifford Peel who was on a troop ship en route to serving in France with the Australian Flying Corps. It is Peel's letter that is generally credited with rousing Flynn's awareness about the possibility of aeroplanes being used to provide medical assistance over great distances. Peel had been studying medicine before the outbreak of war and was keenly interested in the work of the AIM, perhaps envisaging for himself a role in medical missionary work. Peel's letter was startling in its prescience. As usual when Flynn wished to alert the public to a new line of thinking, he used *The Inlander* to publish the letter under the heading 'A Young Australian's Vision'. The remarkable letter reads in part as follows:

> Aviation is still new, but it has set some of us thinking, and
> thinking hard. Perhaps others want to be thinking too. Hence
> these few notes.
>
> **Safety:** The first question to be asked is sure to be 'Is it safe?'
> To the Australian lay mind the thought of flying is accompanied
> by many weird ideas of its danger. True there *are* dangers, which
> in the Inland will be accompanied by the possibility of being
> stranded in the desert without food or water. Yet even with

this disadvantage the only reply to such a query is a decided affirmative. Practically all the flying for the last three years has been military flying, and men have taken, and are taking, risks that will be quite needless in commercial or private aviation in the future; and if we study the records available, and deduct accidents that occurred while the pilot was 'stunting' over enemy territory, we will find that the number of miles flown per misadventure is very large, while the number of accidents per aerodrome per annum is very small.

Difficulties: As in every new adventure there are initial difficulties, so in establishing the aeroplane in the Inland. The first and greatest of these is cost.

Everything is dear by the time it gets Inland, and the question to be settled is: which is the least dear? In this calculation we must reckon time, men, material, and efficiency, in terms of £-s-d.

With aeroplanes I venture to say that, given proper care, the upkeep is relatively light; while the cost of installing compares very favourably – if we realise that to run a train, motor car, lorry, or other vehicle, roads must first be made and then kept in repair, whilst the air needs no such preparation.

The capital expenditure in Europe (according to an eminent English authority) before a motor car can be run is £6,000 per mile, for a train £24,000 per mile, and for an aeroplane about £600 per mile. The problem of overhauls and major repairs present another great difficulty. Most people realise that motor engines require delicate treatment and special machinery when being overhauled. The question of ways and means remains to be solved.

Landing ground may present some difficulties in certain regions, but these will be found where needed.

Machines for Inland work will need to have a large radius of action, say a non-stop run of at least 700 miles, so that the fuel carrying capacity will be large.

Many of these and other difficulties loom very large, as we view them from the distance, but with the progress of aviation, and the more universal use of the motor car, many of them will automatically disappear.

Advantages: ... With a machine doing 90 miles an hour, Darwin is brought within twelve and a half hours of Oodnadatta (excluding stops).

It takes little imagination to see the advantage of this to the mail service, government officials, and business men; while to the frontier settlers it will be an undreamt of boon as regards household supplies, medical attention, and business.

A Scheme: Just by way of a suggestive scheme, I propose to consider that portion of AIM territory east of the Western Australian boundary. In this large tract of land, consisting of one-third of the Australian continent, I am assuming that the bases are situated at Oodnadatta in South Australia, Cloncurry in Queensland and Katherine in the Northern Territory. At the present time these are railheads, hence supplies can be brought up with comparative regularity and minimum cost. From each of these centres the AIM workers can work a district of say 300 miles radius, or an area of 270,000 square miles ...

From Oodnadatta, Alice Springs is about three and a half hour trip. Overland it takes nine DAYS – long ones too.

In the not very distant future, if our church folk only realise the need, I can see a missionary doctor administering to the needs of men and women scattered between Wyndham and Cloncurry, Darwin and Hergott. If the nation can do so much in the days of war surely it will do its 'bit' in the coming days of peace – and here is its chance.'[3]

Peel went on to outline the outlay involved in such a proposal and ended by suggesting that the credit side would accrue from the development of the hinterland by the 'heroes of the Inland'. Flynn's sentiments entirely! Peel's rather cavalier dismissal of financial and other difficulties must have resonated with Flynn who customarily adopted the same approach himself. The letter was a ringing endorsement of the potential of aeroplanes to overcome the distances and isolation of the outback, and fascinating for its appraisal of the fledgling aviation industry. That it came from an aviator gave it all the more credence. Peel was never to know how inspirational he was in the development of Flynn's plans for an aerial medical service. Tragically, he was shot down in aerial combat over France, aged nineteen. In fact, by the time his letter made its way into the pages of *The Inlander* in 1918, his promising young life had already ended. With dreadful irony, aviation, which Peel believed held such promise, was the cause of his death.

Nonetheless, Flynn was charged with enthusiasm about how aeroplanes could be used for the Inland cause. As the war drew to a close, aircraft were being trialled in other parts of the world as mail and passenger carriers and Flynn eagerly seized on these examples as models for how Australia might proceed. The AIM did not have the resources to consider being directly involved at the outset, but Flynn could see no reason why the Defence Department should not use its military aerial force for practical purposes. He suggested that new fliers in training or those needing to maintain their skills could perhaps make themselves useful by conveying doctors and nurses to wherever they were needed – the late 'eagles of war' being employed as 'doves of peace'. Subsequently he broached this subject with the authorities, but while they were sympathetic, they were not yet ready to move. Flynn was always conscious that death travelled so speedily for the Inlanders, while those with the skills to prevent it could not. At least not yet!

Through the next ten years of effort and advocacy, it was Flynn's dogged determination to get a medical service airborne that sustained him and finally resulted in the world's first flying doctor service taking to the skies in 1928. But for now, the plan was only just taking shape.

There was much cajoling, persuading, petitioning and challenging yet to come. It is sometimes easy to overlook the fact that John Flynn was simply a Presbyterian minister, when in fact his entrepreneurial skills, if not his stipend, would not be out of place in boardrooms of today. He had the facility to engage anyone in a discussion of his plans – from the man in the street to the prime minister – and, indeed, had no hesitation in working on both. Dr George Simpson, a great friend to the AIM, described him thus: 'John Flynn, statesman, adroit political strategist – a friend at court in every court. He used his friends as he used himself, he was true to them as he was true to himself.'[4]

A skilled propagandist, Flynn shrewdly realised the value of keeping the public up-to-date with current developments in aviation and whetting their appetites for more – a sort of drip-feed effect. He wanted them to marvel at what aircraft were capable of and to notice how many influential people were also championing their use. He writes gleefully in various outlets:

> A well-known public man, who is interested in the Inland and had read that article by Lieut. Clifford Peel on the possibilities of the aeroplane for service in our regions beyond, wrote in the other day: 'It is a great scheme, and I see no reason why it should not be carried out. My son, who is in the Flying Corps, has written out repeatedly saying that the aeroplane is to be the "distance breaker" for Australia and that no up-to-date pastoralist can afford to be without a machine. They have been rendered absolutely safe, and recent improvements have cut down the consumption of petrol'.[5]

> Captain Harry Butler (AIF), who flew to Minlaton in an aeroplane, against a strong wind, on Wednesday morning, in an hour, returned to Adelaide today in 27 minutes. He flew at an altitude of 17,000 feet, and the distance covered was 65 miles, an average of 144 miles an hour. For us Bushies, the pace of 65 miles an hour is not too bad, but in 27 minutes – well, we would like to

hear the comment of that friend of Mrs Gunn [author of *We of the Never-Never*], who wanted to get out of the country because the neighbours were treading on his corns by approaching within 100 miles of him!'[6]

Even children's letters were mobilised to push the case:

I am waiting impatiently for the time to come when you will be able to start your Inland Air Work, and I will be driving doctors and nurses all over Australia. If I can fly by the time you have your first plane, I would like to be your first pilot. I had a letter from a returned flying man, and he said he thought it would be a long time before commercial aviation would be firmly established in Australia: but that will not hinder your work, and your work will help it. I am going to ____ School at present, but I hope to leave when I am seventeen and go to a flying school.[7]

The AIM Board, although not interested in direct involvement in an aerial medical experiment, were nonetheless persuaded to place a £100 gift from a Singapore banker, Mr C Alma Baker, into a special account in case it should ever be needed for such a purpose. Baker had been in the news during the war when he inspired Australian citizens to gift fifty battle planes to the British government. He had met Flynn by chance on the Albury–Melbourne express and, according to Flynn, wanted to know more about Clifford Peel's ideas. Or was it that Flynn wanted to tell him – given that Flynn never passed up an opportunity to garner support from influential people for his plans! Either way, Baker was interested and, on setting out for Singapore, wrote to Flynn:

The brave pioneers living in these practically uninhabited parts are now entirely cut off from doctors and nurses. None but the men, women and children who live in the Never-Never can

appreciate the great blessing and boon an aerial medical service
will be to them. The people of the Never-Never are the people
who help to keep the big commercial centres together, and those
who live in the big cities and towns of Australia must realise what
these men outback have done, and are doing, for the business of
the community. I think you will find no difficulty, when you
eventually launch your scheme for subscriptions for your aerial
service, in getting the commercial communities of Australia, as
well as the big pastoralists and others, to help finance you in this
very laudable proposition; and on my return to Sydney, at the end
of July, I will have much pleasure in giving you £100 towards
your aerial medical service.[8]

Flynn was aware that the AIM Board had become increasingly
concerned that its superintendent was neglecting spiritual concerns in
favour of more secular ones. So in replying to Baker he was quick to
point out that the board had not launched any such scheme but
assured his supporter that there was a home waiting for the cheque on
his return and that it would be held in trust in case the future
demanded a practical demonstration, 'an air move of our own later
on'. While Flynn was not ostensibly advocating direct AIM involvement – no point in scaring the horses – he was nonetheless privately
harbouring a hope to the contrary. Prior to Peel's death he had guile-
lessly commented: 'Our young friend [Peel] thinks we may do a little
"stunt" on our own account. Perhaps, if he and one of his medical
mates want to prove how easy it really is, we will have a fly just to see!
Why not?'[9]

5

The Elimination
of Dread

. . . .

Flynn now began signalling his interest in wireless communication as an adjunct to an aerial medical service. 'Winged pilots, flying doctors: but they alone cannot save. The bush is at present, for the most part, quite dumb. Not till it becomes vocal in all its parts can it call for the help that has suddenly become so much more mobile than of old. And is there a magic touch that can give the dumb bush its tongue?'[1] Flynn answered his own question, and the answer was 'wireless'. In many respects aviation was less of a problem than the wireless component of the plan. Planes were already in the air and aviation was very much in the news, enjoying the support of disparate groups for a variety of reasons. It would evolve with or without Flynn's engagement. Flynn's role was merely to steer it in his preferred direction – towards an aero-medical application. Not so with wireless. This was much trickier. Flynn's relative ignorance about the way wireless worked enabled him to rather blithely see possibilities where none at that point actually existed. After all, radio was so far the province of the armed forces, merchant ships and hobbyists. It would take every ounce of Flynn's ingenuity and energy to get workable radio sets in outback posts, a development he foreshadowed in 1919, without appreciating how difficult the path ahead would be. Neither did he realise the immense contribution that would be made by a young man named Alfred Traeger who was to invent the pedal radio that ultimately gave the bush its voice.

While keeping the aviation/communication dream alive, Flynn made sure that the nursing arm of the AIM continued its steady pace. By 1919 the number of nursing hostels had increased to five, with one at Flynn's old stamping ground of Beltana added to the total. Present at the opening ceremony was Robert Mitchell, the first Smith of Dunesk missionary, who had presided over the opening of the first hostel in Oodnadatta. The new building was called the Mitchell Home in his honour. 'Flynn's policy with regard to the nursing homes [outlined to the 1920 Federal Assembly] was that ultimately each should become a self-supporting district hospital able to claim government subsidies ... The long-term objective of the nursing arm of the AIM was that, having initiated medical work on the frontiers, it should make itself progressively unnecessary.'[2] This became the process also when the Flying Doctor Service was established. As soon as there was a more appropriate group available to oversee its operation, the Church released it from its jurisdiction.

Flynn was encouraged by the fact that bush people, initially indifferent to the appearance of church workers among them, were now beginning to record a verdict that the AIM was a 'dinkum' force. The presence of nurses and padres in the outback and their willingness to throw in their lot with the Inlanders was having a definite impact. Flynn wanted to add to this positive feeling with a building program that would further confirm the AIM's intention to be a permanent presence in the bush. In 1920 he launched his plans for an ambitious building experiment − a hostel at Alice Springs that would be specially built to overcome the outback aggravations of heat, dust, flies and light. It took six years before the building was finally completed but, when done, it was a model for its time. Its most important feature was an innovative cooling system. Beneath the building was a large cellar from where air was ducted into the rooms. The air entered the cellar from a stone tunnel fitted with wet hessian bags hung from alternate sides that mopped up dust and cooled and freshened the air as it came through. Thick walls, wide verandahs and a raised roof over the central area through which hot air could escape also facilitated climate control during the hot summer months. Gauze on the verandah allowed for sleeping-out accommodation and protection from flies. It was an architectural triumph and still stands today as a museum of local history.

In the 1920 edition of *The Inlander*, along with plans for the Alice Springs Hospital, was a chapter headed 'Sky Doctors'. It gave an account of a doctor in Texas who had invested in a plane, hired a pilot and begun to service a district where the roads were inadequate. 'A real live air doctor' trumpeted Flynn, and a service that had been worked out on a private enterprise basis. Flynn hoped that corporate action would similarly bring succour to the isolated Inlanders of Australia. Also in the chapter was a reference to the aerial feats of Ross and Keith Smith, sons of the saltbush, who had recently completed the first direct flight from England to Australia. Flynn followed the news of these aerial advances with a map of Australia showing where he envisaged sky doctor bases might one day be located throughout the interior. He modestly suggested sixteen – at Burketown, Cloncurry, Longreach, Charleville (Queensland), Bourke, Broken Hill (New South Wales), Port Augusta, Marree, Oodnadatta (South Australia), Kalgoorlie, Mt Magnet, Carnarvon, Port Hedland, Derby, Wyndham (Western Australia) and Katherine (Northern Territory). Each designated base was marked on the map with a miniature aeroplane, and the caption read 'Eventually – Why Not Now?'

Flynn made it sound very simple, dismissing the cost as follows: 'No matter how much it might cost to maintain an individual station, sixteen only for the continent would make no difference in the Nation's annual expenditure – yet would make all the difference in the life's outlook for the brave people of the bush'.[3] Flynn's prophecy of sixteen flying doctor bases would be achieved in 1956, thirty years after this seemingly far-fetched idea was initially promulgated, although not all the bases were in the locations he had foreshadowed.

Flynn often referred to the 'elimination of dread', meaning that if the fear of living in isolation could be removed, pioneers would more readily take their families into the outback. In the 1921 *Inlander* he claimed that there were two great evils arising out this dread:

> Bushmen laugh at risks for themselves, but they mostly stick to their motto 'The bush is no place for a woman'. Hence their temperament suffers. They are great boys, most of them: but when men are deprived of the society of women and children they inevitably miss something in tenderness and brightness. It isn't fair. Also there is an irredeemable loss to the Nation when our most virile, most enduring, most resourceful, most intuitive men remain celibate. Their qualities perish with them, and their race is as if they had not been.[4]

Flynn was convinced that a flying doctor experiment was integral to the elimination of this perennial dread and blamed general apathy for its not getting under way more quickly. He said impatiently, 'We must strenuously spread interest in this reasonable boon for our pioneers, so that it will be granted tomorrow – not next century!'[5]

Flynn firmly believed that isolation and loneliness could kill with the same precision as untreated illness or injury. Stories of great adversity caused by isolation still gained currency and emphasised the need for skilled medical aid to be more readily available. One that Flynn found particularly disturbing was an account by a bushman in western Queensland who had come across four men stricken with fever, alone in an isolated galvanised iron hut. The bushman was horrified to note that the iron of the hut was rattling from the shivering of the sufferers. Flynn bitterly contrasted this story with one involving a sick child who had been fortunate enough to receive swift medical assistance:

> At Iiandia, a sheep station 32 miles from Longreach, the infant
> daughter of the Manager, Mr Jolliff, became seriously ill. Owing
> to heavy rains it was impossible to get out medicine or send the
> little sufferer into town. After communication was established
> with the Aerial Services Ltd., Lieut. McGuinness left for Iiandia
> in one of the company's planes, and the patient and the mother
> were safely landed at a Longreach private hospital in an hour,
> none the worse for their fast trip.[6]

The evacuation had been possible because the Queensland and Northern Territory Aerial Services Ltd, later known as Qantas, had recently been founded by Paul McGinness and Hudson Fysh. Both men had served with the Australian Flying Corps during the war. The service carried passengers, and later mail, over areas in western Queensland.

Flynn met with Fysh for the first time in 1921 and spent hours interrogating him about the possibility of a flying doctor in western Queensland – What type of planes were currently available? How far could they fly? What was their fuel consumption? How did the cost of the purchase of an aircraft compare with leasing? And so on. Fysh was happy to help, astutely recognising that there could be a spin-off for his airline if Flynn were to bring his plans to fruition. Flynn gathered sufficient information from the discussion to report fulsomely in *The Inlander*, quoting Fysh as the source of the opinions and facts, and casually pointing out that Fysh's board was comprised of 'some of the most progressive citizens of that section of the Inland'. Flynn declared with satisfaction:

> Since the commencement of [the Queensland and Northern
> Territory Aerial Services'] preliminary operations in 1920, over

1,000 passengers have been carried, an aggregate of well over 26,000 miles without any mishap except minor damages to the machines. This record should be known to all friends of the Inland. It has already created confidence in aeroplanes out there, and much is expected when real performances begin with running of Aerial Mails, under contract with the Commonwealth Government.[7]

These figures were important because there was still disquiet among the public about whether air travel was entirely safe. To round off the argument, an article from *The Western Australian* of February 1922 was quoted concerning a mercy aerial mission by famous aviator Charles Kingsford Smith, flying for Western Australian Airways, the first airline in Australia:

An interesting indication of the great value of aviation in bringing far away places near to the city and science in case of emergency is a call answered yesterday by Dr Trethowan. The daughter of a resident of Carnarvon recently became very ill, and the services of a skilled surgeon were urgently needed. The case was taken by Dr Trethowan, and the service having been made available following several urgent telegrams, one of the Western Australian Airways machines, flown by Pilot Kingsford Smith, left Perth at 3 o'clock on Tuesday afternoon, and reached Geraldton three and a half hours later. The doctor met the machine there, and yesterday morning left by air at 6 o'clock for Carnarvon, arriving there not long after the town had breakfasted. The needed operation was performed, and by 6.15 last night the Perth surgeon was back at the Geraldton aerodrome concluding what must be the fastest call in his career. It is anticipated that the speed by which the doctor's service was made available by the aeroplane will give the young patient trebled chances of recovery. As it is the story is a splendid instance of the value of aviation in urgent country medical calls.[8]

But despite Flynn's relentless advocacy and supportive articles in the metropolitan press, no benefactor came forward with a cheque big enough to justify the AIM considering an aerial experiment on its own account and there was no tangible interest from governments or the private sector. Undaunted, Flynn continued to seek support wherever he could find it. Pastoralist Sidney Kidman and the rich industrialist Hugh Victor McKay, founder of the Sunshine Harvester Company, both became allies after being on the receiving end of Flynn's enthusiastic public relations efforts. Flynn entertained high hopes for some financial involvement from McKay as McKay had already demonstrated an interest in commercial aviation by backing Norman Brearley who, in Western Australia, established the country's first airline.

And there were champions closer to home. Flynn's sister Rosetta wrote an article in the *Melbourne Herald* claiming the right for all Australians to have access to a range of essential services from mail delivery to medical attention, no matter where they lived and no matter what the cost.

> No one pretends that an aerial medical service will not be a very expensive organisation; but I have heard of it costing the Australian taxpayer £30 to deliver a letter to an isolated fellow countryman outback. And the taxpayer has nothing to say against it, because he has recognised the right of his fellow countryman to have his letter delivered wherever he may be, and whatever it may cost. The letter was probably stuck in a cleft stick by the side of the track and the recipient may have ridden 50 miles to get it, but it was delivered.[9]

She went on to make the point that Dr Holland's expenses in attending Jimmy Darcy, the dying stockman, had amounted to £380. But it would be a cold-hearted person indeed who would seek to assign a price to saving a life.

While Flynn waited for the idea of an aerial service to take hold, the burden of care of Inland people fell to the nursing sisters and patrol padres. Flynn was disappointed that several of the church ministries he had created were vacant, but was encouraged by the continuing success of the nursing arm of the AIM. Two more hospitals were established in 1923, one at the large cattle holding at Victoria River Downs in the Northern Territory and the other at Birdsville in Queensland. Again these came about because of a local crisis.

A nursing home for the isolated centre of Birdsville, so far to the west of Queensland it was almost at the South Australian border, had long been on Flynn's mind. He had earlier earmarked funds for the project but the Birdsville community had decided they wanted a doctor. While they prevaricated, and no doctor was forthcoming, healthy twins born to a bush mother died at three weeks, and the plans for a hostel were hurriedly reinstated. As for the hostel at Victoria River Downs, its appearance was hastened by a malaria epidemic which decimated the station's population. Local contributions of £540 were augmented by double that amount from the federal government. This support had come about unexpectedly, after a party of federal politicians travelling in the service of the North–South Railway Commission had observed at first hand the work of the nursing sisters in some of the hostels and heard heartrending tales of neglect and suffering while at Victoria River. They had encountered Flynn at Beltana at the end of their tour and no doubt Flynn used the opportunity to promote the work of the AIM. Prime Minister Billy Hughes subsequently offered government subsidy to the AIM hostels in the Northern Territory to the tune of £2 for every £1 raised locally. In this and in other ways Hughes had joined the army of Flynn supporters.

Once a nursing home was established, the locals quickly became firm advocates. Ernestine Hill, in *Flying Doctor Calling*, quotes a bushman: 'You had to get a head-rope round a stockman and skull-drag him in to the sisters with a broken thigh, and the next year he'd be riding three hundred and fifty miles off his own bat with a sore finger just to get there.'[10] Such was the spell that the sisters cast, there were tales of old bushies cutting their hair and beards and buying new shirts and blacking for their boots in order to create a good impression when they came calling at the cottage hospital.

In 1924 a unique nursing service began. The managers of four stations in the remote region where the borders of Queensland, South Australia and New South Wales intersect asked Flynn to find them a trained sister who could patrol the whole area. She would make her headquarters at each of the stations in turn and her salary and expenses would be provided. The first of these 'border sisters' was Sister Marjorie Kinnear from Victoria. Using the well-equipped medicine chests which were kept at the stations and travelling by horse, camel buggy or motor transport, Sister Kinnear, with no means of communication other than word-of-mouth, travelled over an area of some 18 130 square kilometres to tend the sick, having the grim responsibility of making diagnoses that only a doctor would normally have to make. Three other nurses came after her and their work became part of bush legend. The last of them, Sister Stewart, became the nursing sister for the Innamincka nursing home when it was eventually established.

Another step was taken a few years later towards the comfort of the Inlanders. While nursing sisters seemed to be ready for service, there was a lapse during the 1920s in the number of patrol padres willing to take up outback chaplaincies, a situation which led one woman to write: 'From a woman's point of view, you can't help wishing we had more travelling padres in the Inland, especially when you see and hear of men who have "borne the heat of the day" and are working beyond their strength. It makes a woman wish she were a man for once. Surely it is no hardship, but a privilege, to have two or three years in the Inland.'[11]

Perhaps the sisters had a slightly easier time of it in that they had, in the hostel, somewhere to call home. There was no such luxury for the padres who were constantly on the move, staying in rented lodgings during their brief sojourns between patrols. So it was decided to instigate a system of two-man patrols to give relief from the strain of the long, lonely journeys, the first being established in 1927 for the west Queensland and Gulf area. In addition, motor vehicles began to replace the horses and camels that had hitherto been the patrol padres' main method of transport. This was made possible because increasing motor traffic had made tracks more navigable, particularly in the dry months. Flynn was a staunch advocate of this new arrangement, having himself known the hardship of the solitary traveller. 'Mechanical breakdowns are inevitable at times, and their repair often necessitates four hands, not to mention two heads. In that country, also, sickness often smites hard and sudden – and one cannot drive one's car along a narrow track when one's head is swimming!'[12]

While motor vehicles were becoming more and more useful, Flynn's determination to also drive home the point about aviation as a means of transport was apparent in the 1924 edition of *The Inlander*. Hitherto, the magazine had featured a string of camels plodding across the bottom of its cover. Now the camels were joined by a motor vehicle piled high with boxes and baggage and a plane soaring overhead. But while the transport issue was throbbing with life, the issue of communication was desperately in need of a kick-start.

6

An Aerial Medical
Experiment

. . . .

In 1925 Flynn began initial wireless experiments on a field trip with
George Towns, a wireless expert. Their primitive equipment was
tested at various places and eventually word got back to Flynn that
their messages had been picked up at remote stations and also in
Adelaide, Melbourne and Sydney. Although numerous problems were
encountered on the experimental trip, the first phase of the wireless
experiment at least established that anyone with a car for a power
source and sufficient funds for equipment could have a voice in the
bush. Refining the process so that a workable transmission set would
be accessible to those with limited means and expertise was still a long
way off. The experiments terminated at Alice Springs and Towns
returned to Adelaide. Flynn stayed in Alice Springs for the next nine
months, ostensibly to work on the construction of the hospital. But
there was another motive. The AIM Board were becoming increasingly critical of Flynn's devoting so much time and energy to the
wireless project, surely outside the AIM's realm of interest. In lying
low, and keeping away from head office and the rumblings of the board,
Flynn hoped to deflect attention from his non-spiritual activities. The

nursing home total received an extra boost that year, when in addition
to Alice Springs, hostels were established at Lake Grace and Marble
Bar at the request of the West Australian Government.

His pleasure at the completion of the Alice Springs hospital was
tinged with gloom when Flynn learned that his old ally, Hugh Victor
McKay, had died. Andrew Barber, arriving with the official party to
open the hospital, brought the sad tidings. However, along with news
of McKay's death came the advice that he had left a bequest towards
an aerial medical experiment. Would this be the financial backing for
which Flynn had waited so long? No longer reluctant to face his
colleagues, he hurried back to Melbourne to determine the nature of
McKay's beneficence. McKay, always a supporter of Flynn and his
ideas, had remained faithful to the last with a sum of £2000 towards
an aerial experiment, provided additional financial support came from
other quarters. Given that McKay died a millionaire, presumably he
could well have afforded to provide whatever additional amount was
required. But as an astute businessman, perhaps he saw some merit in
forcing a level of commitment from others. There was no better way
of rallying people behind a cause than to have them take responsibility for its financing. Whatever the reason, the gift was intensely
appreciated, for without it the Flying Doctor Service may have taken
even longer to become airborne. The dream was on its way to becoming a practical proposition when the Federal Assembly formally
authorised the AIM Board to take all necessary steps towards an aerial
experiment. How sweetly this directive must have rung in Flynn's ears.

An Aerial Medical Service Advisory Committee was formed
in 1927 whose membership included prominent representatives of
aviation, medical, wireless and pastoral interests. Flynn chose these
people with care, knowing that an expert team would be needed to
satisfy the requirements of the various bodies that would have a stake
in the service. The Department of Civil Aviation, the British Medical
Association and the Postmaster General's Department all had regulations that would demand compliance. Approval would have to be

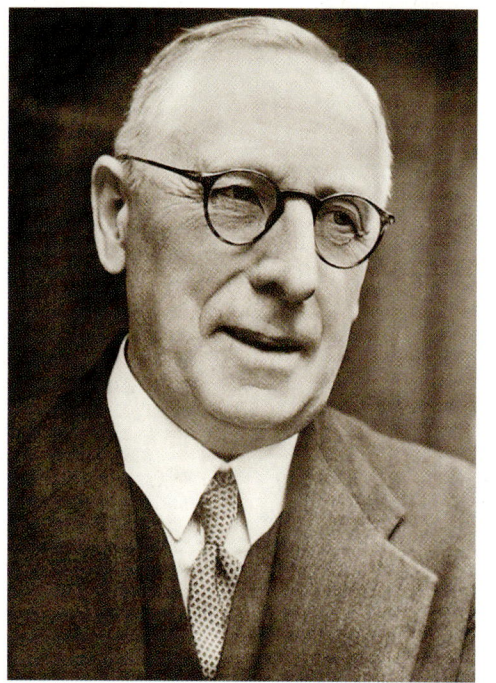

The Reverend John Flynn

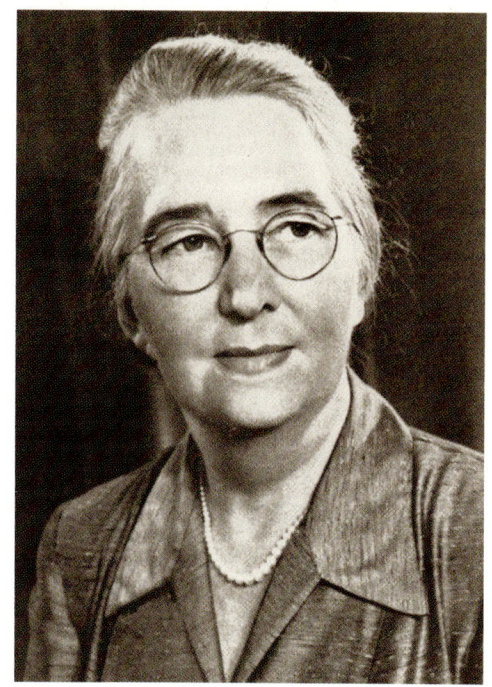

Mrs Jean Flynn

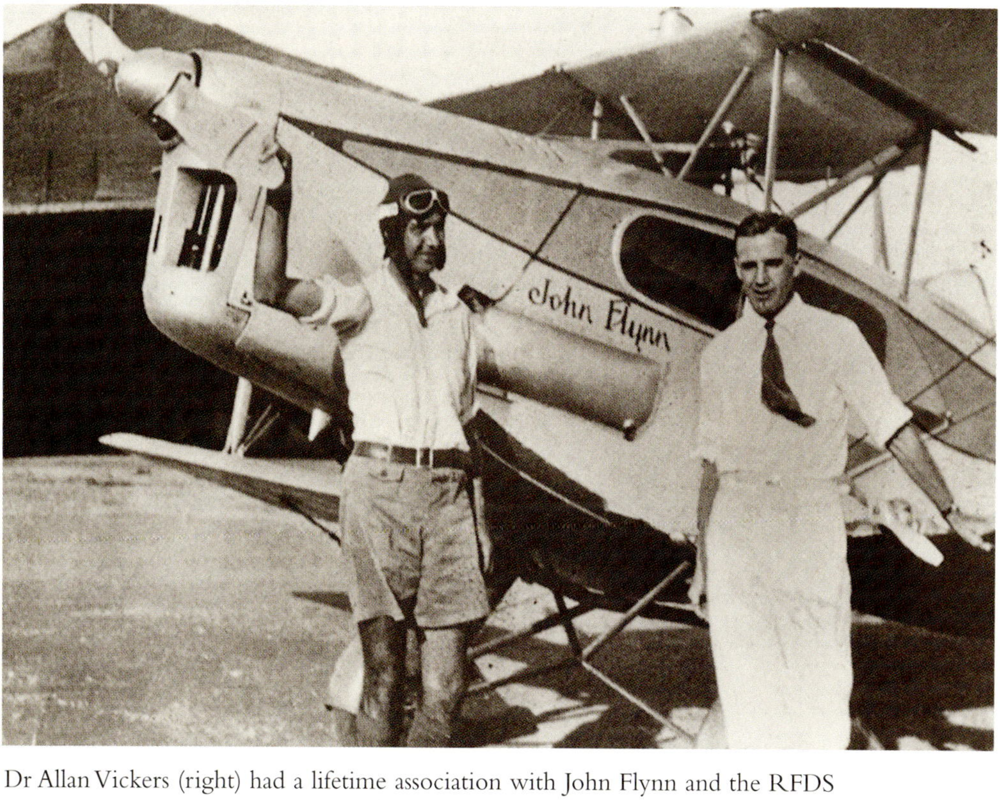

Dr Allan Vickers (right) had a lifetime association with John Flynn and the RFDS

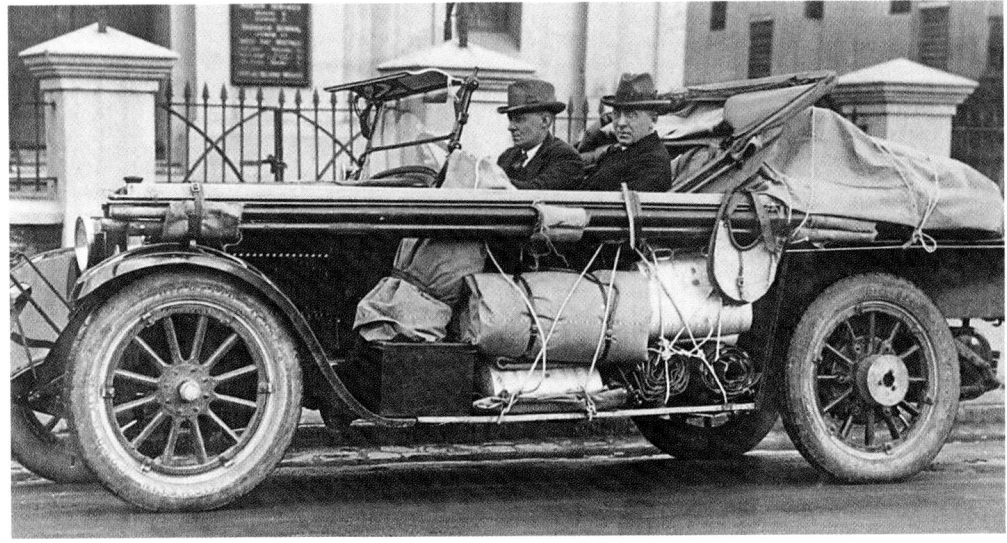

John Flynn (in the passenger seat) and George Towns (wireless expert) start out on a radio field trip in the heavily loaded Dodge buckboard in 1925

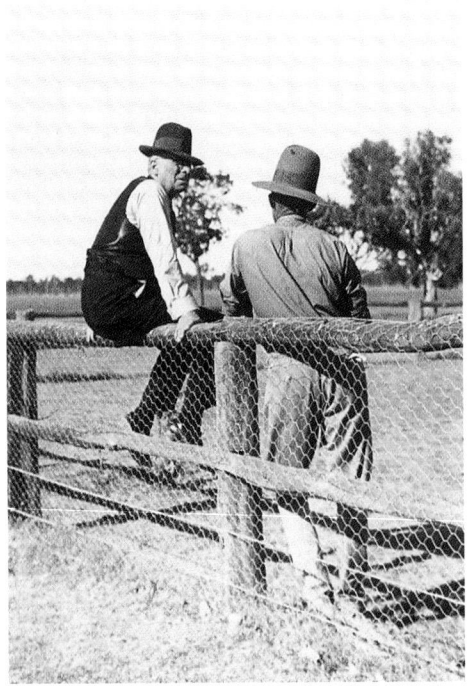

Flynn yarning with a bushman

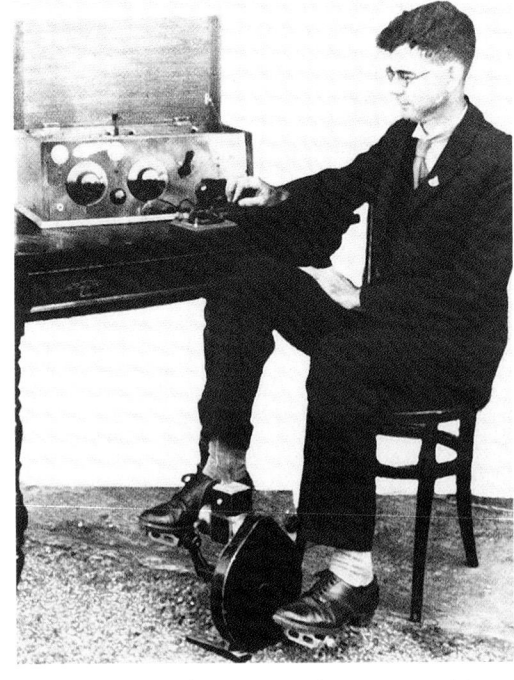

Radio expert Alfred Traeger demonstrates his pedal transceiver in 1929

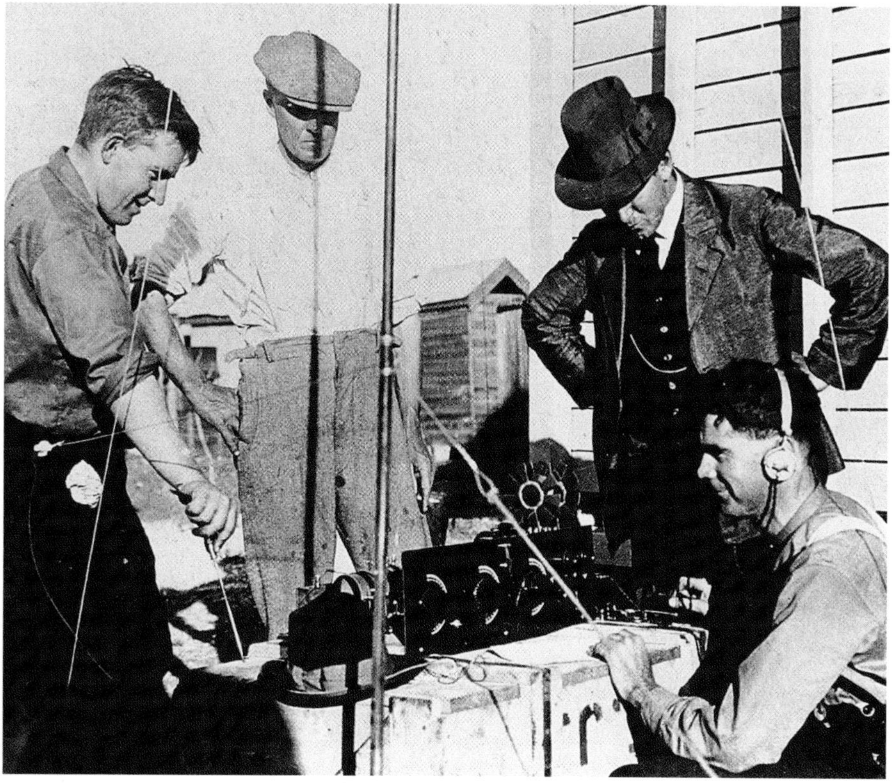

Traeger (seated) transmitting a morse code message at Cloncurry in 1928 before an admiring audience. From left: George Towns, Ernest Gollan, Padre George Scott.

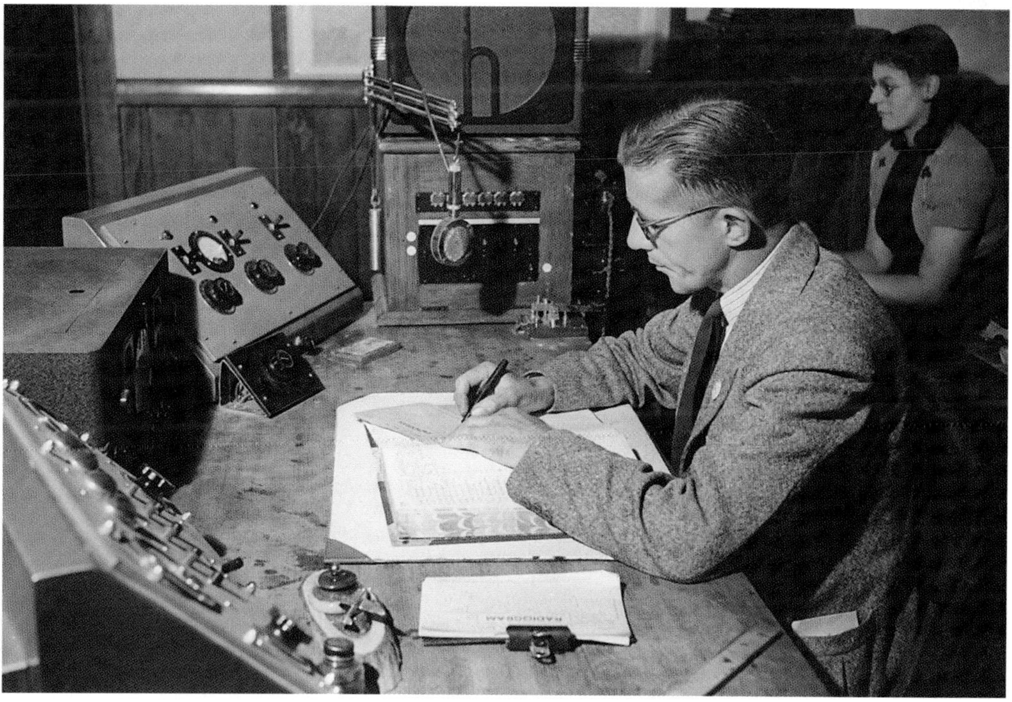

Frank Basden, a legendary figure in the outback radio system

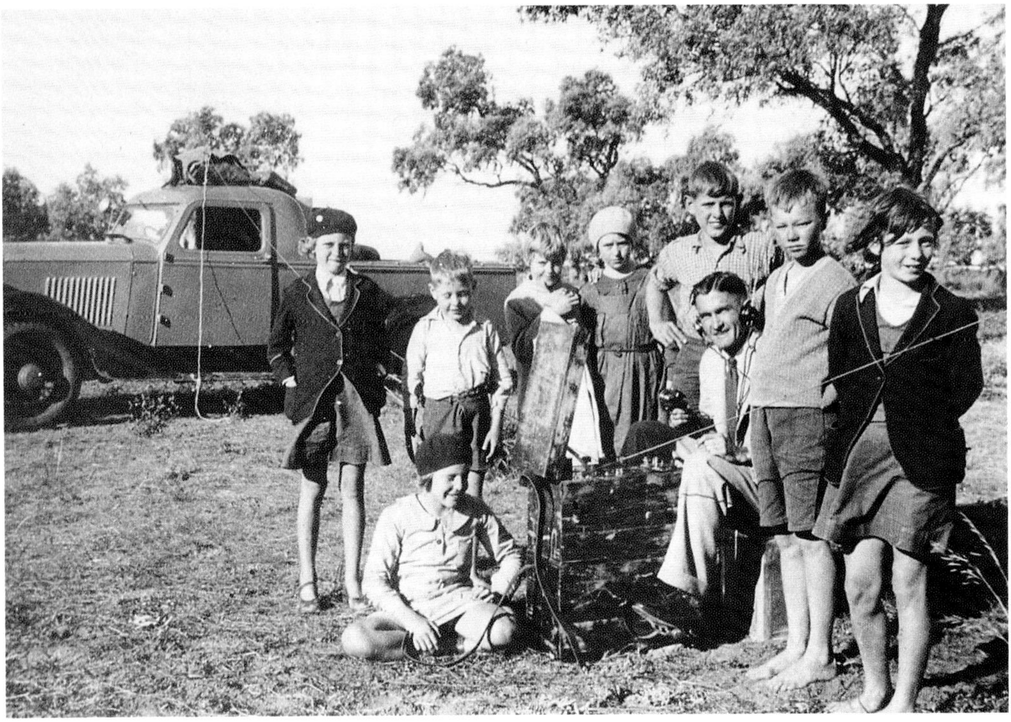

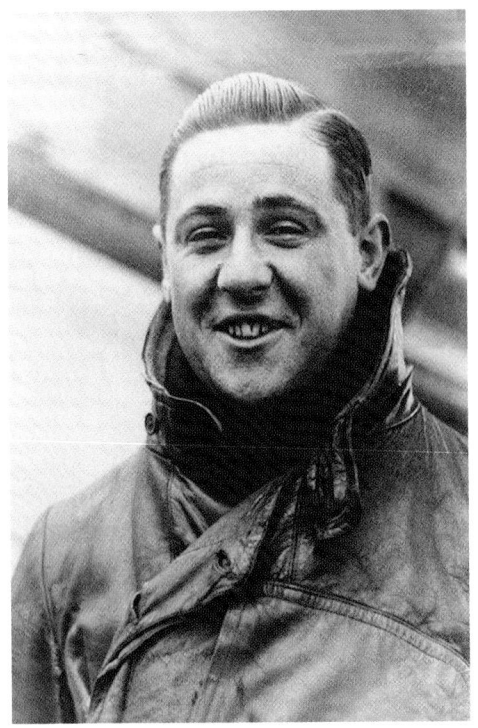

Patrol padre, Rev. Fred McKay, in touch with Cloncurry base while taking bush children to the coast for a seaside holiday

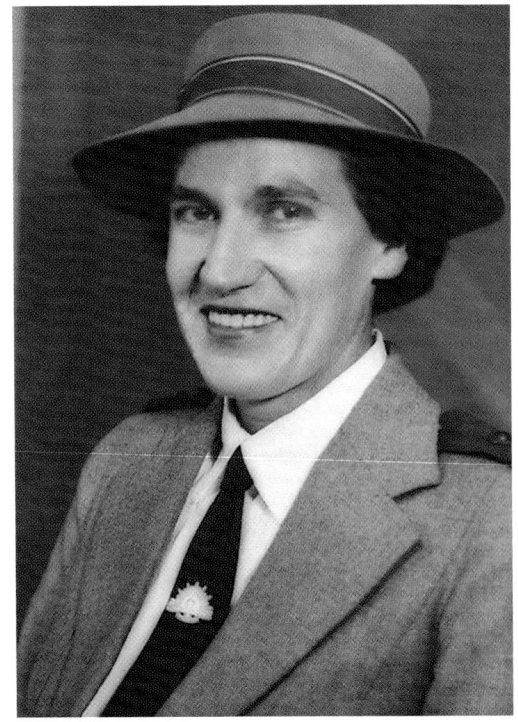

Arthur Affleck, first RFDS pilot

Myra Blanch, first flying sister to be formally employed by the RFDS at Broken Hill in 1945

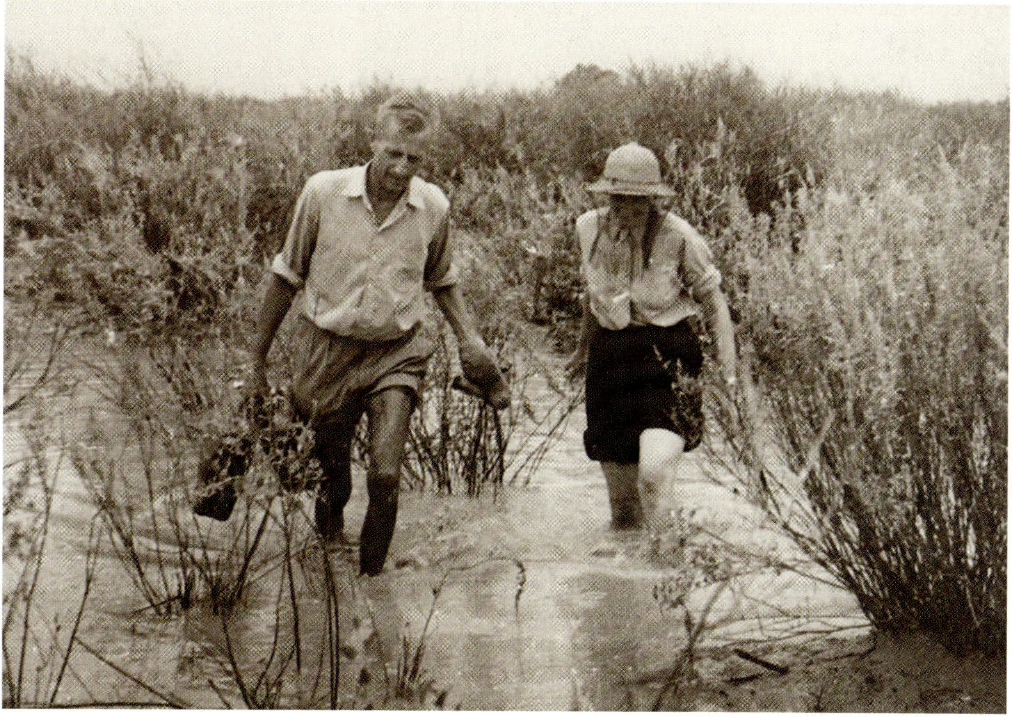

Reaching patients was not easy for Sister Myra Blanch and Dr John Woods

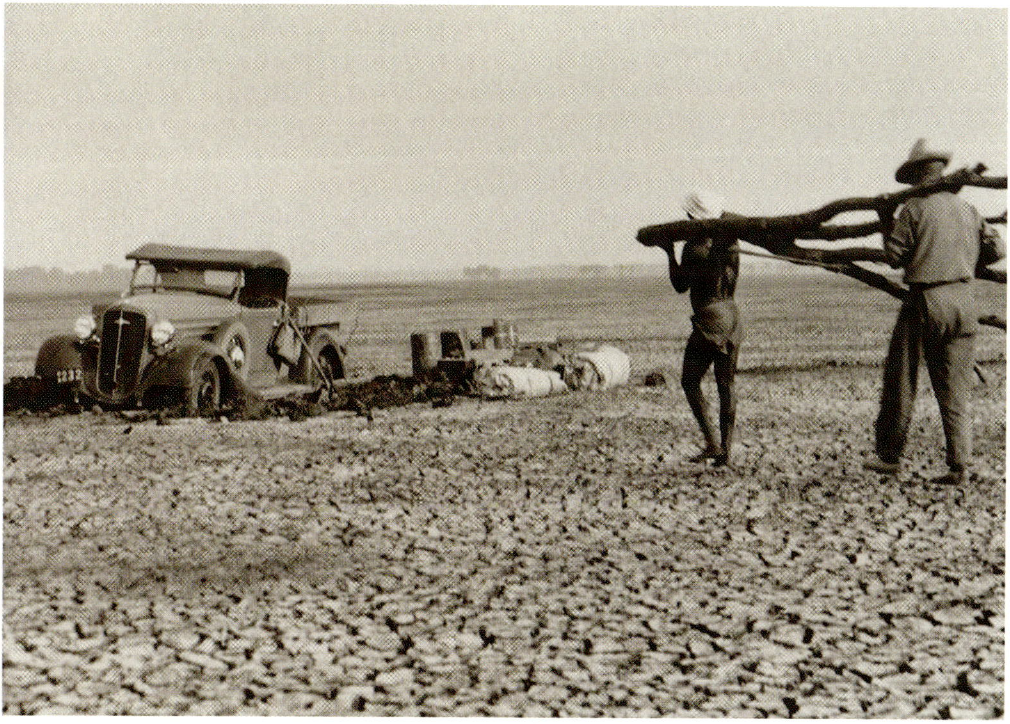

Driving in remote areas could be very slow and hazardous. Here a Ford truck is stuck in the outback.

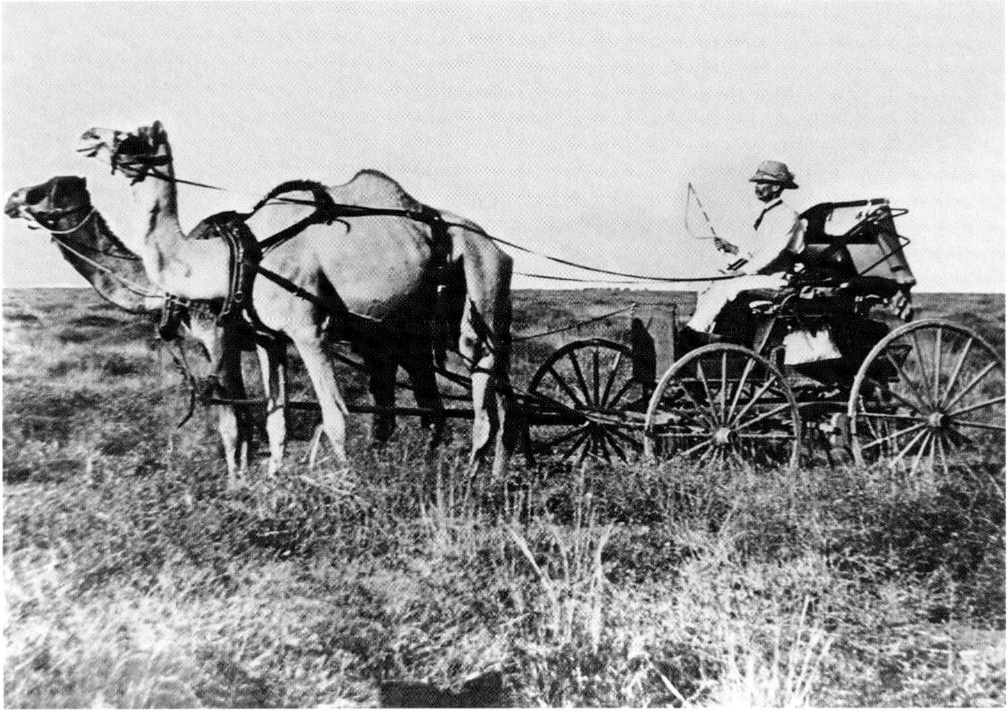

The Rev. Jim Stevens patrolling the Pilbara in Western Australia in 1913

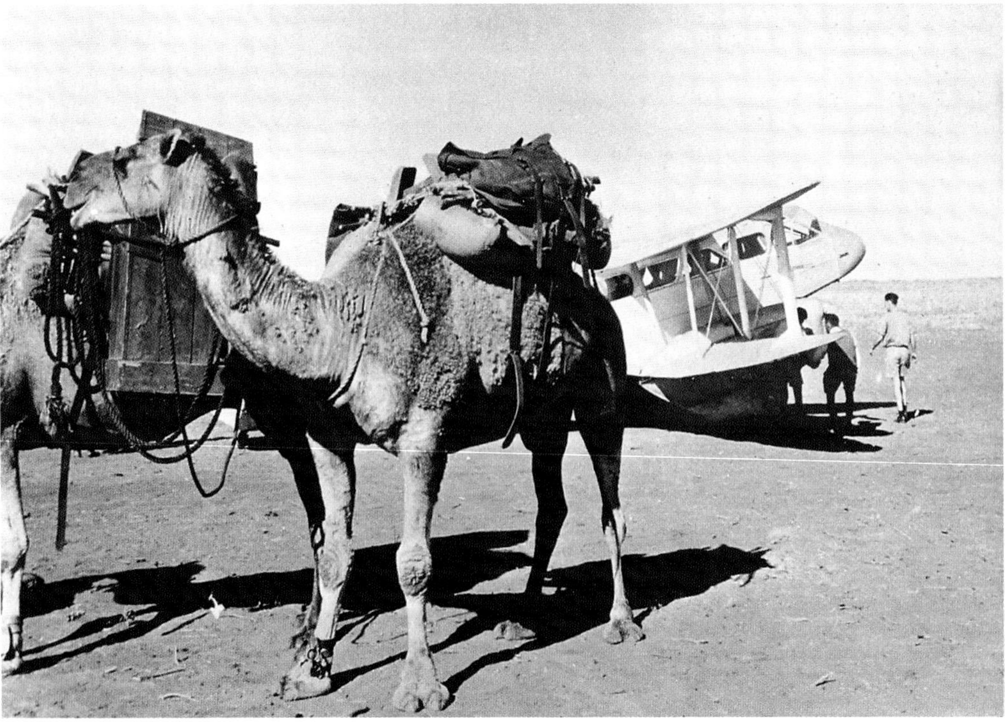

In the early days of the Flying Doctor Service camels were used to transport fuel and essential supplies to where the planes would land

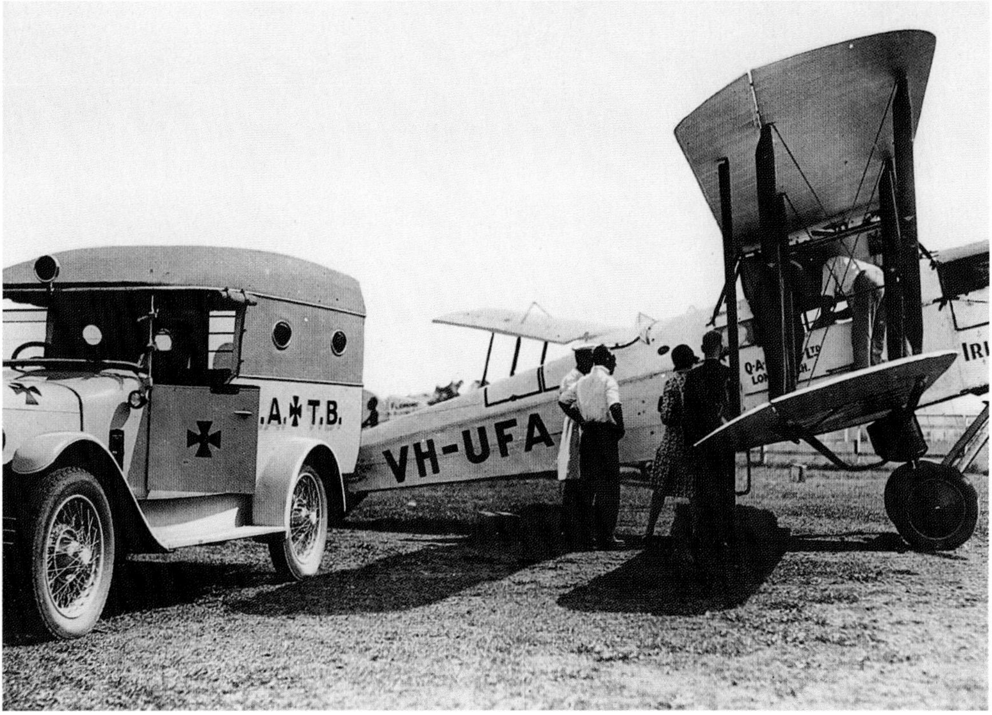

A patient in the early 1930s is transferred from the flying doctor plane to a waiting ambulance

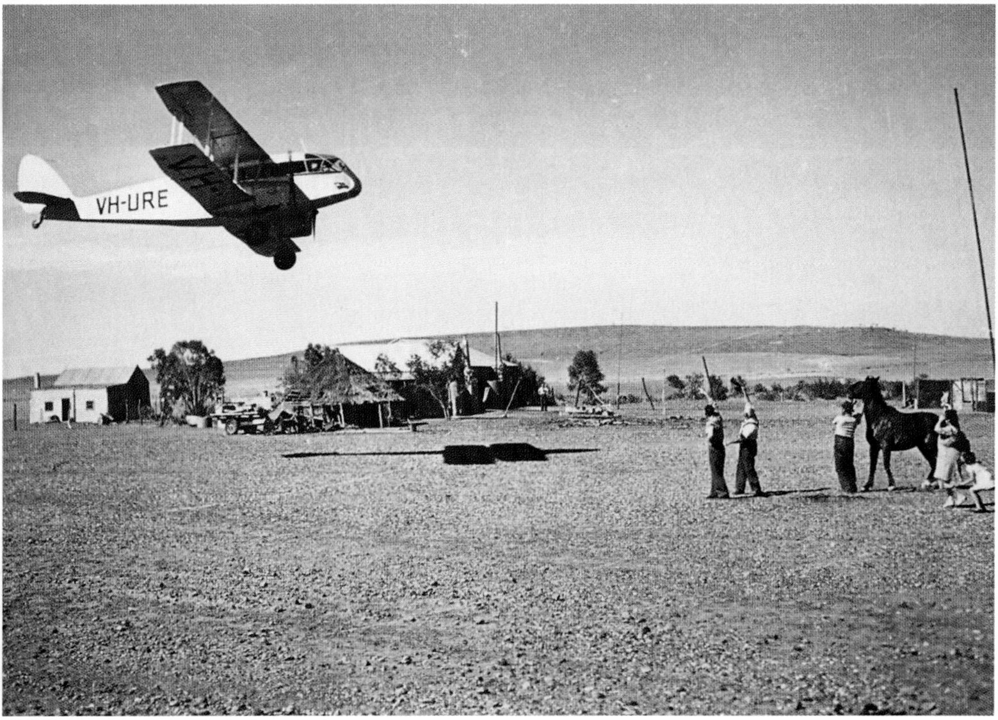

A Dragon aircraft flies over an isolated homestead

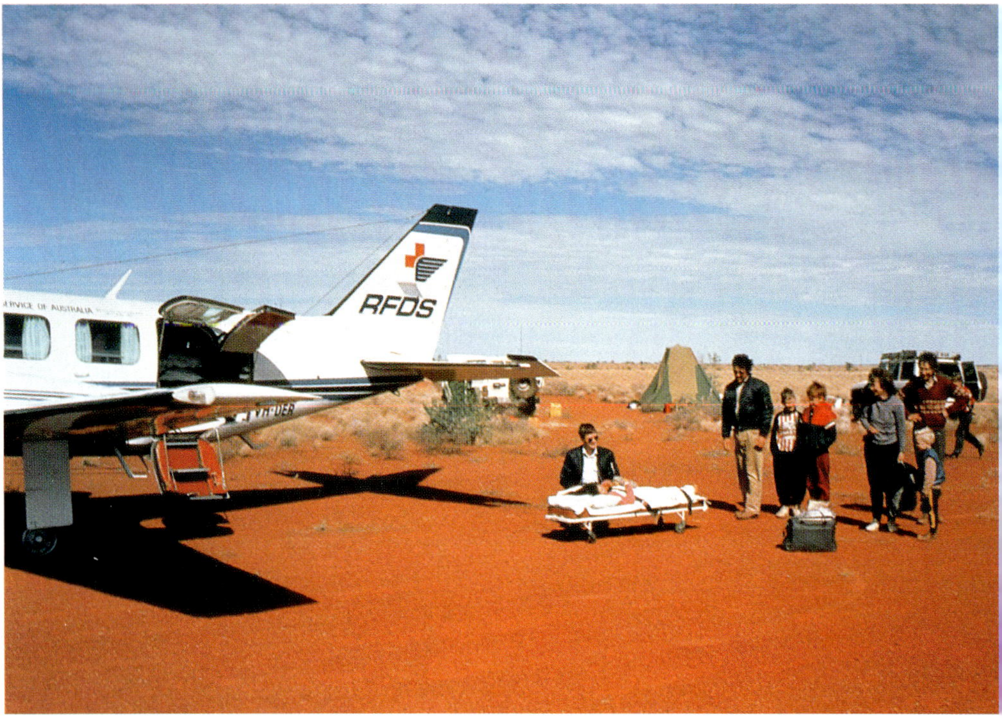

An evacuation after an accident on the Canning Stock route

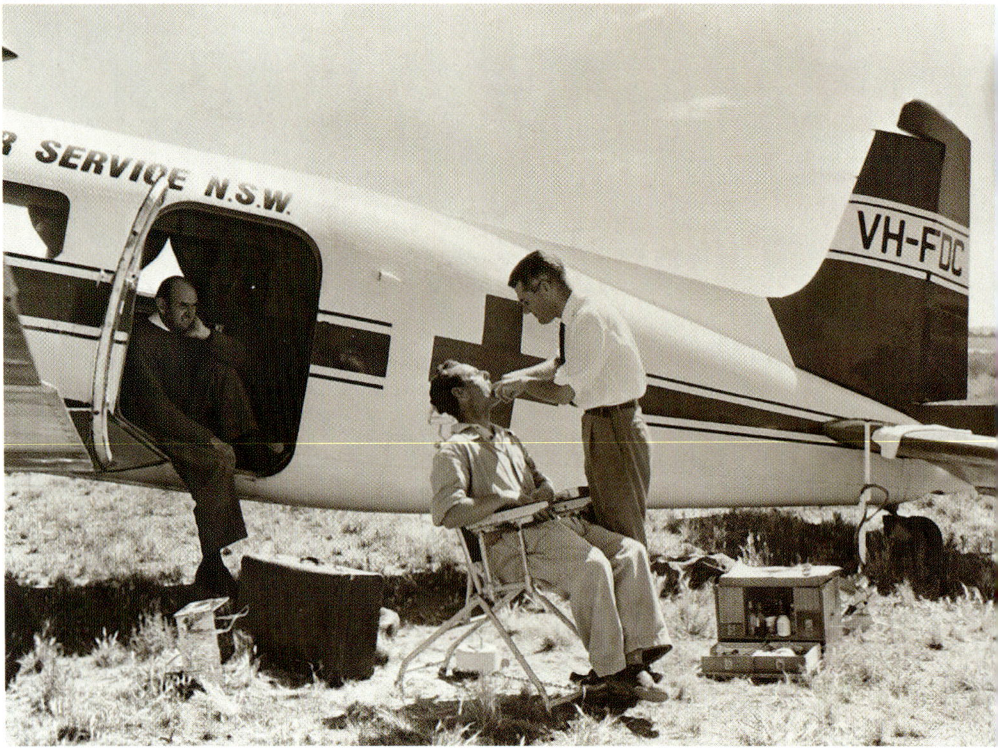

A flying dentist in the 1960s works on a patient in an outdoor surgery gained from the state government of whichever centre was chosen for the experiment. And the residents themselves would need to be willing. The time for talking and promoting was over. Now was time for real action and the task ahead was massive.

Seven thousand pounds was the amount thought necessary to finance a doctor and equipment for one year. Andrew Barber, Flynn's collaborator on *The Bushman's Companion* and a faithful friend to his plans, had joined the AIM earlier in 1927 as patrol organiser and now became chief fundraiser for the aerial service. In addition to the £2000 from the McKay Trust, £5000 had still to be raised. The Wool Brokers' Association of Australia, conscious of the benefit of the scheme to pastoralists, contributed £1000, as did the Civil Aviation Department. Smaller amounts were also received from various parties. But there was still a slight shortfall. Dr George Simpson, Flynn's chief medical adviser for the aerial medical experiment, explained the source of this final amount: 'When time was running out and the appeal was still five hundred pounds short of the target, John Flynn and Mr Barber gave a joint personal guarantee to put everything in order. Mr Barber laughingly said, "That was all right for John Flynn, he didn't have £500".'[1] It was not the first time that Flynn had dipped into his own pocket when 'rations', as Flynn termed them, were needed.

A number of sites had been suggested as the base of the first aerial operation, including Broken Hill, Broome, Port Hedland and Carnarvon. Ultimately all were rejected in favour of Cloncurry which became the first beneficiary of the service for a number of reasons. Its 480-kilometre radius brought it within striking distance of Cape York Peninsula, west into the Northern Territory and south almost to South Australia, areas all desperately short of medical resources. The necessary wireless network was not yet developed but there was an existing telegraphic system and a skeleton telephone system in the area of operation by which help could be summoned by those in need. There was an aerodrome to receive patients and a forty-bed hospital to which they could be conveyed, where there was a resident medical officer and a full nursing staff. The Queensland Ambulance Transport Brigade was already in existence and would work in concert with the aerial service attending to patients within a closer range while the flying doctor service attended to those further removed. And there were sufficient numbers in the Cloncurry area to allow for data to be accumulated about what facilities would be needed when the rest of Australia joined the program.

However, before the final decision was made on Cloncurry, Flynn wanted a thorough investigation made of the area to evaluate conditions, disseminate information about the impending service and to garner support. Andrew Barber, with George Simpson as medical adviser and motor mechanic, set out on a three-month exploratory trip in June 1927 from Adelaide to Darwin and into western Queensland. It was an arduous journey. The roads were poor and punished motor vehicles mercilessly. Simpson had his hands full replacing parts and mending punctures. In addition to servicing the vehicle, Simpson spent gruelling hours extricating it from bogs. The upside of the trip was that the two men enjoyed many examples of bush hospitality and time and again were reminded of how important a part the AIM organisation played in maintaining the health and welfare of outback life. As they travelled Simpson attended to medical needs, Barber to spiritual – and both attended to the promotion of the aerial medical service.

When they arrived at Alice Springs they saw the hospital which had been completed the year before and described the building as 'imposing'. In a letter to his mother, Simpson gave an arresting description of what he saw:

> The hostel is the centre of the town, and the general meeting-place for all. Everyone takes an interest in the place, which they appreciate as their own. Funnily enough, here the two men in the district who were most opposed to the hostel at first were the first patients, and now are most loyal and enthusiastic supporters.

It is great, too, the way the AIM nurses are welcomed everywhere
they go, and the interest all bushmen take in them. They do a
great work, and the AIM does great things for the Inland. Alice
Springs hostel is a model of what the AIM can do. Two fine
wards, electric light, sewerage, good living rooms, wide verandah,
and everything possible for comfort and convenience. As I sit on
the open verandah, looking towards the Gap, I feel I am almost in
a different world to yours. A tame emu is walking about outside.
Blacks are playing about their camp, and a string of camels is
coming along the road laden with goods from Oodnadatta.[2]

On reaching Cloncurry, Barber described it as 'a fine place, about
1700 inhabitants and 5000 billy goats'. Simpson was more expansive:

Cloncurry is a fine inland town, but like many another, it has seen
better days. It is a junction town – railway junction, airway junction, roadway junction. It is situated at the junction of hilly mining
country and the fine pastoral plains extending east round Julia
Creek. At one time there were 14 hotels in Cloncurry, and all
full. Many have been burnt, unfortunately (they were covered by
insurance), but there are still some quite fine ones left. There are
several wide streets, shops, garages, churches, etc. The hospital is a
couple of miles out of town; so is the aerodrome; so is the Chinese
market garden. Planes fly north to Normanton on the gulf, west
to Mt Isa and Camooweal, and south-east to Longreach once a
week. The Normanton plane returns with live fish from the gulf,
and once a week we have fresh sea fish 200 miles from the coast.[3]

Providentially, from a propaganda point of view, a call came for
Qantas several days after their arrival to send a plane to Mt Isa to
evacuate a patient who had fallen down a mine shaft and fractured his
pelvis and spine. Simpson accompanied pilot Norman Evans, watched
over the stricken man on the return flight, and delivered him safely to

the local hospital. Simpson found it fascinating to soar swiftly and easily over country that he and Barber had just covered so slowly and painfully by car. Barber wrote about the event as follows: 'The road route is about 156 miles; the air route is 124 miles. The plane just took one hour to fly in. This case will help Dr Simpson in many ways to report fully on this whole question of travel by air. The patient said the journey by air was less worrying to him than the trip by ambulance of about 134 miles from hangar to hospital.'[4] It was a dramatic enactment of the way the aerial service was destined to operate.

Barber and Simpson reported from their trip that the outback was most emphatically in need of the sort of facilities that an aerial medical service could provide. Armed with this intelligence, Flynn submitted a draft proposal to the Advisory Committee that was adopted as the charter for the world's first flying doctor service. The objective would be to provide an aerial medical service operating from Cloncurry to outback districts, thus linking them with existing ambulance and hospital services. The one-year experiment would commence about Easter 1928. The service would operate over a 480-kilometre radius except for those inaccessible areas where suitable landing grounds were not yet available. Said Flynn in *The Inlander*, 'It is probable that a mantle of comparative safety will be cast over an area exceeding a quarter of a million square miles'. He continued triumphantly, 'Have you taken that in? More than 250,000 square miles!!!'[5] Flynn had reason for such elation. After years of toil, of painstaking recruitment of supporters, of bearing disappointments with composure and of fighting his detractors, he had been vindicated completely.

Flynn's efforts to interest Hudson Fysh in his plans had borne fruit. Qantas agreed to charter to the AIM a DH50 aeroplane which had been fitted out to carry a stretcher. It was decided that the best policy for the present was to buy flying miles from an established aviation company rather than the Aerial Medical Service (AMS) owning, servicing and piloting their own plane. The AIM would pay Qantas two shillings per air mile flown. The Commonwealth Government at last came to the party with an offer of a subsidy of one shilling per mile up to 25 000 miles flown, thus underwriting half the expenses of the operation. The AIM would be liable for ten pence per mile for any unflown mileage. It was a satisfactory arrangement for all parties. The plane would be called *Victory* for obvious reasons, but also to honour benefactor, Victor McKay. Arthur Affleck, one of Qantas's best pilots, was assigned to the aerial service. Dr Kenyon St Vincent Welch was the outstanding candidate from a number who had applied for the job as the first flying doctor. Welch had been unable to serve in the war and was keen to make a contribution to his country, even though it meant leaving behind a wife, children and a thriving medical practice in Sydney.

The duties of the doctor would be threefold: to attend accident and other urgent cases, rendering first aid on the spot and transporting the patient to the nearest hospital if necessary; to make periodical medical tours to districts beyond the range of existing services; and to be available, when other duties permitted, for consultation for isolated local doctors.

Aware that his experiments with wireless transmitters were still in their formative stage, Flynn undertook to continue the research with a view to enabling those who were destitute of telegraphic facilities to eventually be able to call for aid. He pointed out that unless the problem with communication was solved, further extensions of the AMS would be pointless. This was a courageous statement as it locked him in to a definite timeframe for resolution of the wireless dilemma. He further pointed out that although there were sufficient monetary reserves at present, additional funds would be needed if the service were to continue beyond its experimental year. 'Will-makers please note', wrote Flynn cheerfully. Subtlety was out of place at this critical stage.

When the first AMS flight took off on 17 May 1928, Flynn knew that he was well on his way to giving people the sense of security that would encourage them to populate the interior and infuse new life into the dead heart of the continent.

A ringing endorsement of the aerial service was given by Dr Welch in his first month's report:

> On the 24 May, 11 am, came a call from Dajarra, 108 miles
> south-west. As the plane could not land at Dajarra, it was
> necessary to take a trip of 200 miles by rail motor, leaving at
> 5 pm and arriving at 11 pm. The patient was elderly, with
> pneumonia, and not amenable to treatment of any use, but the
> relatives were comforted by the visit, and I spent until 12.30 am
> seeing other people with minor ailments. We arrived here
> [Cloncurry] again at 6 am, very cold and stiff. The rail motor is
> a little open truck, and you sit on a petrol case. There is no wind
> screen, and the wind goes hard in the 'wee sma' hours. We had
> close calls with numerous stock on the line, and finally hit a large
> kangaroo full and square – he was dazzled by the headlight. It
> nearly upset the truck. Last week the truck did come to grief in
> a collision with a horse. THE PLANE IS SAFER![6]

At the end of the experimental year it was agreed that the ideal aimed at had in great measure been attained. There had been some disappointments and shortcomings, such as periods of inactivity for the doctor, flights that were made when unnecessary and a certain amount of clashing with existing services. In addition the AIM had been obliged to pay over £400 for unflown mileage, the shortfall between the 25 000 miles contracted for and the number actually flown. But the organisers saw these as merely pointing the way to a more efficient performance in the future and approved a second-year trial.

During his one-year tour of duty, Dr Welch made fifty flights, covered a total of 20 000 miles, saw about 250 patients and held fifty consultations with local doctors. He visited twenty-six different centres and on only one occasion was not able to answer a call owing to weather conditions. (Alternative arrangements were made.) With great relish, the Rev. Barber reported on Dr Welch's schedule: 'He makes a two-hundred-mile flight before breakfast, operates and sees patients, and returns to his base for lunch. Next day perhaps he is called a couple of hundred miles in the opposite direction. Distance is eliminated – miles mean nothing.'[7] The jaunty tone speaks volumes for the satisfaction all participants must have felt that the scourge of distance had finally been eradicated, at least in the area around Cloncurry.

Flynn was not present to see the culmination of the first year's activities. He had been persuaded to take twelve months furlough, his first break in sixteen years. Flynn was a man of simple tastes – he had never owned a home, nor did he value the accumulation of possessions. He had never hesitated to divert portions of his own modest salary to AIM concerns, like buying radio components. Aware of this, friends and colleagues all over Australia secretly contributed £666 for an overseas holiday fund, and Flynn set off on a trip to Europe, Canada and America. In London he was surprised to learn that he had been appointed as an Australian delegate to the First International Health Aviation Conference to be held in Paris. While there he began to realise how widespread his reputation was and found his advice and opinions eagerly sought by delegates from many countries in Europe, Asia and America. Wherever he went, he amassed documents, maps, newspaper articles and information that might prove useful for the Inland cause. He returned home refreshed and eager to find out first hand how events had progressed in his absence. Before going overseas he had been aware that Alfred Traeger, the wireless expert, had perfected a pedal radio set suitable for use in the bush that could send messages in morse code and receive replies by voice transmission. While Flynn was overseas, Traeger had installed a base station in Cloncurry with a handful of transceivers positioned within its range of operation. On his return Flynn was delighted to learn at first hand from Traeger and Dr Atcheson Spalding (Welch's replacement as flying doctor) that both the radio network and the AMS were performing to expectations.

7

A National Movement

. . . .

By 1930 all interested parties were convinced that the aerial medical experiment should be continued and an extension of the service to other centres would be justified. Flynn began to marshal his ideas for the service to go national. Unfortunately, the onset of the Depression caused the AIM Board to stay its hand and Cloncurry continued to be the only base in operation. During the subsequent Depression years, Australia's economy suffered a huge downturn – wages were cut, government expenditure reduced, interest rates lowered, and taxation increased. Unemployment peaked at 32 per cent. Governments, both state and federal, were in a state of flux.[1] In this climate an expansionist policy for the AMS could only be regarded as imprudent. With many financial demands on the public purse, the federal government cancelled its subsidy to the AMS, and private contributions dwindled. However, the Queensland government, grateful for the service being rendered to the Queensland outback, was convinced that the service should continue, and provided a subsidy of £800 per annum. Notwithstanding this support, the AIM still had to make up the shortfall, and the Flying Doctor Service found itself struggling for survival. It was fortunate that Flynn had been unremitting in his push for an aerial medical service. Had he let matters take their own course without prodding from behind, the Depression must surely have put paid to the scheme altogether. Even so, drastic measures were called for. Qantas was persuaded to reduce their mileage charges, the number of flying days were curtailed and Flynn and other paid staff of the AIM and AMS took salary cuts to demonstrate their commitment to the project.

During the early years of the Depression, Flynn's publicity machine received an unexpected boost with the publication of Ion Idriess's book *Flynn of the Inland*. With a certain amount of poetic licence, Idriess painted a romantic picture of the AIM and outback life. As a result Flynn achieved almost legendary status, a position that caused him some discomfort but one he tolerated for the sake of the increased interest in the work of the AIM that resulted.

Also fortuitous was a meeting that took place between Flynn and Dr Allan Vickers. Vickers had been one of the original applicants for the role of first flying doctor, and drifted once more into Flynn's orbit just as Flynn was looking for a new doctor for Cloncurry. In referring to Flynn's character, *The Presbyterian Messenger* had earlier asked: 'Was there ever such an agitator as Mr Flynn? He never wearied, and never ceased from talking up and interesting others in his schemes. He would button-hole a man – any man who would listen – and would lay his plans before him with an earnestness as if he expected that one to finance the whole undertaking. Then he would go from him and begin it all over again with the next person he happened to run against.'[2] The full force of these persuasive powers was turned on Vickers, and before long, Vickers had agreed to abandon his planned study trip to London and head north to Cloncurry.

Vickers brought to the role of flying doctor not only his medical expertise but also a dapper appearance and a charismatic personality, traits which were useful for Flynn's publicity push. Indeed, one of Vickers' epic mercy flights brought him Australia-wide coverage in the press. It involved a Croydon publican who was severely injured when a kerosene refrigerator exploded. Years later, the Rev. Fred McKay (who succeeded Flynn as superintendent of the AIM) gave this account in the *Frontier News*:

> Pneumonic complications set in before Vickers got [the injured man] to Normanton, so it was a case of a race against death to get him to Brisbane, more than 1000 miles away. Vickers, with pilot Eric Donaldson, flew through a heatwave of 122 degrees, battling against heavy headwinds at 80 knots in the old DH50. The mother of the patient sat on the only seat. Dr Vickers, open-shirted and busy, was perched on an empty kerosene tin beside the half-conscious patient. They stopped at Cloncurry, Winton and Longreach. About 140 miles from Brisbane the man died. The flares of Archerfield came up in the dark. The plane landed like a weary albatross after a long and tiring flight. Reporters and photographers rushed up to it. The headlines came out next morning. Death had won the 1300-mile race.[3]

Despite the tragic outcome, the event focused attention on the difficulties inherent in the running of the Flying Doctor Service. Flynn knew that accounts like these would be useful in galvanising support. He recognised in Vickers a man who could serve the AMS in other ways, as well as medically. In early 1933, he persuaded a rather reluctant Vickers to embark on a lecture and fundraising tour. After a shaky start, Vickers found his feet and his talks detailing the work of the AMS and recounting anecdotes about mercy flights undertaken in extreme conditions, like the Croydon one, won the approval and admiration of the crowds. Using a selection of slides to accompany his talks, Vickers addressed church groups, schools, clubs and social service groups, and gave interviews to press gatherings and on radio. The resultant publicity was enormous and donations once more began to flow. The high point came when Flynn and Vickers were invited to address federal parliament. This was a golden opportunity. If they could put their case persuasively, the government might be moved to reinstate the subsidy they had withdrawn when the Depression first began to bite. Vickers and Flynn gave a compelling performance, and by the end of the session, the federal government was back on the financial bandwagon.

The time was now ripe for Flynn to re-visit his plan to turn the Flying Doctor Service into a national organisation to bring medical aid to all the sparsely settled regions of the continent – over five million square kilometres. Flynn had come to the realisation that it would be impracticable for the Presbyterian Church, through the AIM, to undertake the unlimited liabilities and responsibilities of extending these services throughout such an enormous area. The plan was ambitious – to create five Flying Doctor bases in addition to the inaugural Cloncurry base. Flynn knew it would not be as simple as his earlier work, setting up one nursing home after another. As with Cloncurry it would need the support of a series of organisations and the assistance of state governments. To this end, Flynn set his sights on the Premiers' Conference to be held in June that year. When the conference took place, the response from the premiers to his bold proposal was encouraging and a motion was carried giving tentative approval to a nationwide aerial medical service.

Flynn then set to work to draw up a detailed constitution that would serve the new organisation. His only misgiving was whether he could persuade the Church to relinquish control of the air service at a time when it was receiving positive press and bringing great credit to the AIM. It was a curious position for Flynn to find himself in given that the AIM had not always been fully supportive of the time, energy and finance necessary to keep the AMS afloat. But parochial concerns gave way to a broader vision and in September 1933 the General Assembly of Australia authorised the AIM Board 'to assist in creating a new organisation of national character, to establish and maintain Aerial Medical Services adequate for the isolated areas of the continent'.[4]

With this hurdle overcome, in February 1934 the new national organisation, re-named the 'Australian Aerial Medical Service' (AAMS) was formed and the Victorian Section inaugurated in some haste in order to report to the next Premiers' Conference due to meet that month. There was a long and sympathetic discussion among the various premiers, all of whom pledged support in various ways. A particularly resounding endorsement came from the Queensland Premier who said: '"Flynn of the Inland", as you know him, established his first unit in the Cloncurry district, and has conferred incalculable benefit on outback pioneers, upon whom we depend for the development of this country. Queensland, Western Australia, and the Northern Territory depend largely on this form of medical service. I have no hesitation in saying that its worth to Queensland is ten times the sum of money expended by the Government on it.'[5]

The premiers' deliberations resulted in the following resolution: 'That this conference approves of a general co-operation of the Governments and the States with a view to furthering the Australian Aerial Medical Scheme.'[6] Flynn's initial program, begun in a relatively small way in Cloncurry was on its way to becoming an organisation of national standing. Each subsequent section of the air service would be independent and administer its own affairs with a federal council supplying liaison with the federal government. This was important if the AAMS was to continue to attract federal funding.

The fledgling plan for the first flying doctor base in Cloncurry had taken many years to come to maturity. Once the AAMS was formed the next four bases came comparatively quickly. As the smallest mainland state, Victoria had no need for a flying doctor service on its own account, but decided instead to sponsor a base at Wyndham in the far north-western corner of Australia. It began in July 1935 with an aeroplane, the *Dunbar Hooper*, under charter from MacRobertson Miller Airways. Included in the Wyndham base's area was Halls Creek, the scene so many years before of Jimmy Darcy's demise. Ironically, it was to Halls Creek that the new flying doctor, Ralph Cato, made his first mercy flight. Further, one of the chief supporters of the establishment of the West Australian bases was Dr James Holland, Darcy's medical benefactor.

The structure of the Victorian Section was used as a prototype for the other mainland sections. The mantle of safety was extended three months later to Port Hedland, under the auspices of the Western Australia Section, with Allan Vickers, now finished his service at Cloncurry, as the flying doctor. Alf Traeger set up the radio bases for both. Broken Hill followed in 1937, the first base to be administered by the New South Wales Section, in a Fox Moth chartered from Australian National Airways (ANA). The Eastern Goldfields Section inaugurated the fifth base in 1938 in Kalgoorlie, taking over the work of the private aerial ambulance service operating from that city. Norma King in her history of the section, *Wings Over the Goldfields*, says that even though the local service was working well, it was considered time 'to join the AAMS and become affiliated with the recently formed Federal Council and receive a share of its financial benefits'.[7] This move relieved the pressure on the Western Australia Section which had been faced with the huge task of servicing the largest mainland state.

A sub-base was also established at Normanton in the Gulf country to minister to areas out of the range of the Cloncurry base. Dr Jean White, who was medical officer for Normanton and Croydon, filled the role of flying doctor in addition to her other duties.

Flynn now turned his attention to establishing a sixth base at Alice Springs. An organisation had been set up in South Australia to raise funds to commemorate the work of the pioneer women of that state. Flynn approached its president, Adelaide Miethke, intent on persuading her that the funds her group had earmarked for a 'flying sister' at Port Augusta would be better employed in underwriting a flying doctor base at Alice Springs. As told to author Harry Hudson by Adelaide Miethke herself, Flynn put up a convincing argument:

> Without wasting time on preliminaries, he launched into his
> subject. He spread a large map of Australia on the floor, and within
> minutes [we] were on our knees poring over it. Flynn pointed to
> Cloncurry and indicated the range of that Base by putting his
> thumb there, and described a circle with outstretched palm and

fingers. He did the same with Wyndham, Port Hedland, Kalgoorlie
and Broken Hill; then he pointed to Alice Springs. "Here," he said,
"we have nothing! All this great area and no medical service.
Look! Put a Base *here*, at Alice Springs! We could cover four
hundred miles all around it, this way, that way and that. We just
need that Central Base to complete the Mantle of Safety".[8]

Once more Flynn's prodigious powers of persuasion paid off.
Miethke was converted to the flying doctor base proposal and £5000
was subsequently handed over. The base in Alice Springs began
operation in 1939. This was not the only service Adelaide Miethke
rendered to the people of the outback. She was later instrumental in
utilising the Flying Doctor radio network to form the famous School
of the Air which began in Alice Springs in 1951.

Throughout this time Flynn, the elder statesman of the AAMS,
and his various hard-working and dedicated deputies, continued to
run the federalisation campaign. Their efforts were rewarded in 1936
when a meeting in Melbourne moved that the Federal Council of the
AAMS be formed, composed of two representatives from each
section. It would be an umbrella body to link the various sections,
coordinate all activities and establish contact with concerned federal
government departments and negotiate federal funding. (The Federal
Council is now called the Australian Council.)

It was not until 1939, after some frustrating delays, that the
Queensland Section was formed, and the AIM transferred control of
the Cloncurry base to the AAMS and the Normanton base was
closed. Also transferred were the land, building and wireless plant at
Cloncurry as a free gift, together with a cash donation of £1000
towards immediate running expenses. This marked the end of AIM
involvement in the direct running and financing of the Flying Doctor
Service and the maintenance of the wireless stations and was the culmination of Flynn's plan to give all states in mainland Australia a stake
in the service.

In 1941, the organisation decided to adopt the title 'Flying Doctor Service' by which it had become generally known. In 1955 Queen Elizabeth granted the use of the prefix 'Royal'.

During the eleven years of AIM control, from 1928 to 1939, the flying doctors covered 319 834 flying miles without an accident, except for one occasion when the doctor and pilot were missing for five days owing to the plane making a forced landing during a cyclonic storm.

The cost to the AIM of maintaining both flying doctor and wireless services during the eleven years was £46 830, apart from the considerable indirect services provided by the AIM office staff, and the patrol padres who installed and serviced many of the pedal sets.[9]

Flynn had married his long-serving secretary Jean Baird in 1932 when he was fifty-one years old. Without children of his own Flynn always regarded the aerial medical service project as his child and often spoke of it as such. He supported and nurtured it, and when its development was complete, like a good parent he sent it out into the wider world. And so the AMS moved from the auspices of the Presbyterian Church to a wider arena. It had come of age.

In relinquishing its control, the AIM was not abrogating its interest in the well-being of the Inlanders. Attention was still paid to the recruitment of patrol padres, the building of nursing homes and the continuation of other welfare work it had inaugurated, all designed to bring comfort and support to the Inlanders. In 1980 the AIM took on the title 'Frontier Services', a name Flynn himself had often informally used to denote the nature of the work, and to this day continues to care for bush people challenged by the problems of distance.

Again and again, Flynn was vindicated in his belief that what Inlanders needed most was to feel protected against the reality of isolation and the possibility of untended illness and injury. This letter illustrates:

> As a resident of the Cloncurry district for many years ... I would like to say a few words of praise for the AIM and the good work

it has done and is still doing. The pleasure, comfort and feeling of security that the AIM, with its ambulance plane and flying doctor gives to the women and children outback, is beyond description, and I am sure I am expressing the thoughts of thousands who receive these benefits when I say that it would be a great pity to change the existing order of things. The amicable relations between Qantas Airways, the AIM with its ambulance plane, doctors, and careful, efficient and reliable pilots – with special mention of Dr St Vincent Welch, the first flying doctor in the Cloncurry district, who did splendid work – have greatly helped to make the outback parts of Queensland much better parts to live in.[10]

In 1939 Australia was once again at war and in succeeding years further development of the Flying Doctor Service was curtailed as resources were diverted elsewhere. Flynn was appointed Moderator-General of the Presbyterian Church, a move which brought great satisfaction to Flynn's supporters all over Australia. He placed the AIM on a war footing and put its various resources – nurses, patrol padres and the wireless network – at the disposal of the government. Some AIM buildings became troop hospitals or were used as homes for army nurses. Flynn organised an Inter-Church Welfare Club in 1940 as a recreational centre in Darwin for the troops stationed there. Staffing shortages meant that concessions had to be made to Flynn's policy in the Flying Doctor Service of 'one man, one job', that is, that doctors should not pilot planes. With the relaxation of this rule Dr Harold Dicks in Western Australia became the first flying doctor to pilot his own plane. And flying doctors attended to patients at army outposts in their localities as well as to their usual patients.

In 1940 the Presbyterian College at McGill University in Montreal in Canada conferred an honorary doctorate of divinity on Flynn. From that point on he was often referred to as 'Dr Flynn', fitting perhaps, given his relentless pursuit of a better medical deal for the bush.

During the war and in succeeding years, Flynn revisited each of his old stamping grounds doing what he did best – encouraging, supporting, guiding, inspiring. He was now in his sixties but age had not wearied him. He created further welfare projects like the Old Timers' Homes in Alice Springs where old bushmen could see out their declining years in an appropriate environment. From 1939 the AIM had ceased to have any direct responsibility for the administration of the Flying Doctor Service but Flynn's interest in the organisation never abated and he served on both the federal and state councils.

John Flynn attended what was to be his last Flying Doctor Council meeting in May 1950; he died of cancer the following year. His body was cremated and his ashes flown to Alice Springs by the Commonwealth Government and interred in the shadow of Mount Gillen. As Flynn lived in the hearts of the outback people, so his ashes were laid to rest in the heart of the outback. At the memorial service on 23 May 1951, a huge crowd – clergy of all persuasions, bush men and women, AIM nurses, past and present members of the Flying Doctor Service – gathered to honour an exceptional man. Fittingly, hundreds more, from the most remote stations and settlements throughout the Inland, tuned into the service on the Flying Doctor radio network. Central Australian patrol padre Kingsley 'Skipper' Partridge was chosen to deliver the address and said of John Flynn: 'Here he worked with pride and joy in a task well done. So here he lies where he longed to be. He is not dead; his work abides; his memory is forever eloquent. For across the lonely places of the land he planted kindness, and from the hearts of those who call those places home, he gathered love.'[11]

In 1935 Flynn had persuaded a young Queenslander, Fred McKay, fresh from his ordination into the Presbyterian Church, to sign on with the AIM and become patrol padre for the Birdsville region. They had first talked in 1934 when McKay was stationed at the Presbyterian Church at Southport in Queensland. McKay was a lifesaver in his spare time and in an SBS television program entitled *Sacred Stones*, the 92-year-old Fred McKay told the story of sitting on the beach with

Flynn, McKay in a swimming costume, Flynn in his customary tie and waistcoat. McKay recalled Flynn's words: 'We have to build a hospital at Birdsville. I'm looking for a young bloke who's game enough to go to Birdsville'. McKay absentmindedly played with the sand as they talked, prompting Flynn to say, 'Fred, the sand out at Birdsville is a lot lovelier than this.' McKay noted that it was typical of Flynn not to state directly what he wanted but the message was clear, and sure enough, McKay went to Birdsville, influenced as many had been before him, by the power of John Flynn's conviction. As the two men set off along the beach to the dressing shed, Flynn strode ahead with his long strides. 'I walked behind him', said McKay, 'and I tried to put my footsteps in the marks he was making. I often say that from that moment, my steps were in his footsteps all my life'.[12] McKay carried out his work with great dedication and became, like Flynn, a well-loved figure. He was a popular choice as superintendent of the AIM after Flynn's death, a position he held until 1974. One of his first tasks was to help with the re-building of the Birdsville hospital which had been destroyed by fire. As Flynn had with the building of the hostel at Alice Springs, McKay also knew the value of a hands-on approach. A loyal friend to the RFDS, Fred McKay served as AIM representative on the Federal Council from 1951 until 1973 and as a councillor of the New South Wales Section (later named the South Eastern Section) from 1952 until his death in 2000.

Flynn's widow, Jean, had expressed a desire for a distinctive stone to be placed above her husband's burial place to symbolise a bush grave and Fred McKay was keen to carry out her wishes. When no suitable rock was found in the nearby MacDonnell Ranges, the search contin-ued to the desert near Tennant Creek, 400 kilometres north of Alice Springs. Here was Karlu Karlu, an Aboriginal sacred site known to Europeans as the Devils Marbles, which years before George Simpson had described as 'gigantic granite stones balancing on one another, and worn by wind and weather into perfect spheres'.[13] One of these imposing boulders was selected and transported to the grave site.

On 12 August 1953 it was lifted on to the stone plinth of Flynn's grave and a short service was conducted by Fred McKay in the presence of his wife and Jean Flynn. When Jean Flynn died in 1976, her ashes were laid to rest with those of her husband.

Throughout the entire time that John Flynn presided over the AIM, a church building had never been erected in its name. All available funds had always been spent on the building of hostels and other practical expressions of his solicitude for the well-being of the Inlanders. Led by Fred McKay, Flynn's supporters and admirers decided that a fitting memorial to the life and work of the father of the Flying Doctor Service would be a non-denominational church in Alice Springs. On 5 May 1956, five years to the day after his death, the John Flynn Memorial Church was opened. This honoured Flynn's wish, expressed in the early 1920s, that one day a cathedral would be built in Alice Springs where services would be 'attended' by a congregation of thousands listening in via a radio network stretching over the whole of Central Australia.[14]

Flynn was often the centre of controversy during his life and in death not less so. In 1996 the Warumungu and Kaytetye peoples, traditional owners of Karlu Karlu, requested that the rock above Flynn's grave be returned to its place of origin. This outraged many of Flynn's supporters who thought that such an act would be tantamount to desecration of a Christian sacred site. Protracted negotiations took place over the ensuing years, and were finally resolved when the Arrernte people of Alice Springs, as a gesture of respect for John Flynn, offered a sacred stone from their own land as a replacement. At a ceremony on 4 September 1999, the rocks were exchanged. All parties concerned came to regard the event as a powerful act of reconciliation of which Flynn himself would have thoroughly approved.

The satisfaction of looking back over a lifetime and knowing that everything planned has been accomplished falls to the lot of few people. But it happened for John Flynn – not through chance but because he worked assiduously throughout a long career to make each of his dreams a reality. He was a pathfinder — with a rare ability to embrace the technological developments of his age in order to harness them for a humanitarian cause; and he served this cause faithfully. At the time of his death his mantle of safety was securely positioned over the interior with thirteen AIM hospitals, a boundary-riding ministry which numbered seven motorised patrols, eight flying doctor bases and a radio network that spelt the end of isolation for the Inlanders. The dread had been eliminated.

TRAEGER: THE PEDAL RADIO MAN

8

Sending and Receiving

. . . .

In the annals of the RFDS the name of pedal radio man Alfred Traeger is writ large. Without the contribution of this shy self-effacing radio engineer, John Flynn's vision of creating a communication system to underpin the Flying Doctor Service may have been severely compromised, a fact acknowledged by Flynn when he said, 'Without a wireless transmitting station at every isolated habitation, an Aerial Medical Service would be 75% futile.'[1] This claim was made well before Traeger had developed a means of efficiently generating power for the transceivers so it was a courageous statement. In making it, Flynn was virtually admitting that his grand plan would be doomed if the aviation and radio concepts could not be made to work in concert.

Flynn was aware of radio as a necessary corollary to aviation almost as soon as he began to develop the idea of a flying doctor. But when the Flying Doctor Service formally began in Cloncurry in 1928, the problem of how to achieve a quick and effective means of signalling for help had still to be resolved.

Flynn began to dabble in radio himself when it became apparent that the type of set he had in mind for the Inland wasn't yet on anyone's drawing board. He sought advice from radio hobbyists and pored

over textbooks and wireless magazines trying to increase his understanding of this new technology. After persuading the AIM Board
to invest in some wireless equipment, he began experimenting in his
spare time, pulling apart components and reassembling them in an
attempt to unlock their secrets. It was not a task for the faint-hearted
but Flynn was never that. Bearing in mind that wireless receiving sets
had only just started to make their way into city homes, where there
were existing power supplies, Flynn's vision of a set for the outback
that could receive *and* transmit without a readily available power
source (few homes in the bush generated their own) was a big ask. To
add to the complications he wanted the set to be small, portable,
cheap, able to withstand rough handling, and simple enough to be
operated by amateurs. And there had to be a central base station with
which the small sets could communicate. An ambitious scheme such
as this was bound to have its detractors but it is a mark of the man that
he refused to be discouraged. In fact, Flynn's radio-learning curve was
so dramatic that it took him from rank amateur to Honorary Life
Member of Radio Engineers Australia in 1947 for his efforts in connection with the development of inland communications.

With the aviation aspect of the plan gathering momentum, it had
been Flynn's intention to begin an assault on the radio problem during
1926 but the plan was hastened when he was introduced to George
Towns, who volunteered six months of his time in an honorary
capacity to help launch the program. Towns had the right credentials
for the job. He had spent years in the outback so was familiar with the
territory, plus he had served with a wireless unit during the First
World War. Flynn accepted his offer with alacrity. The objective was
to establish whether wireless transmission was feasible over a large
distance using the rudimentary apparatus that had so far been cobbled
together. The tests were to take place at Beltana, Innamincka,
Birdsville, Marree, Oodnadatta and Alice Springs. Flynn acquired a
Dodge buckboard for the trip which was custom fitted to take their
mass of equipment.

In addition to Towns, Flynn was fortunate in having other supporters keen to assist. Dr George Simpson, the son of a Presbyterian church elder and an avid AIM supporter, had six weeks to fill in before taking up a position as a surgeon on a ship leaving for England from Adelaide. Simpson was not only a medical man but also a proficient mechanic so volunteered to acquaint Flynn with the workings of the Dodge engine. As it was mandatory for motorists to know how to effect running repairs if stranded in the bush, Flynn was grateful for the instruction. Ernest Fisk, managing director of Amalgamated Wireless Australia (AWA) donated equipment. Radio engineer Harry Kauper offered his workshop in Adelaide and undertook to stay alert for any radio messages that might successfully emanate from the trials that Flynn and Towns were to conduct in the field. Simpson, Fisk and Kauper were among the many people who came under Flynn's spell and who would continue to contribute to the AIM effort.

Before setting out for Beltana, Flynn and Towns spent a couple of months in Adelaide assembling their transmitting and receiving equipment. They came up with the idea of powering the equipment with a generator run off Flynn's car engine. Mounting the generator on the splashboard on the passenger side of the vehicle, they jacked up the back wheel, and ran a belt and pulley arrangement from the wheel to the generator. Unwieldy but workable. But the generator was not strong enough to deliver a steady voltage. Ever helpful, Harry Kauper advised Flynn to visit a young electrician named Alfred Traeger who had made a high voltage generator that might suit their purpose. Flynn went to Traeger's workplace and negotiated the purchase of the generator out of his own pocket. Having secured the generator he rushed back to the workshop, little realising the significance of this chance meeting – that he and Traeger were destined to form a partnership which would ultimately solve the problem of communication in the Inland.

Traeger's generator proved a workable replacement. With the addition to the equipment of a 12-metre aerial (made of light metal tubing in four sections) strapped to the side of the Dodge, and a block and tackle to erect it, Flynn and Towns were at last ready to set out. Their mobile station had been licensed by the Postmaster General's Department and given the call sign 8AC.

Month after gruelling month of testing followed. Each test involved unpacking and assembling heavy equipment, erecting the aerial, jacking up the car for power and painstakingly testing the apparatus for telephony and morse. Transmission over long distances was not successful during the day so Flynn and Towns were forced to carry out their experimentation in the freezing desert temperatures of evening and early morning. Progress along the track was sometimes achingly slow. Flynn reported on one occasion covering a distance of only a few hundred metres over an eight-hour period when the heavily laden Dodge became trapped in sand. Visits to the various nursing homes along the way were bright spots in the journey and Towns was able to provide entertainment with his powerful receiving set that picked up programs from the newly formed broadcasting stations on the coast. Flynn saw this as a useful way to familiarise people with radio and interest them in its capabilities. It was an inspirational and unusual experience for the people of Cordillo Downs, in the extreme north of South Australia, to be able to join with the congregation of St Paul's Cathedral in Melbourne in hymn singing. Thus there were triumphs along the way but also a lot of heartache. The trip ended in Alice Springs. Towns had to return to Sydney and Flynn was needed for the construction of the hostel.

Describing the experiments in an article for a 1927 edition of *Wireless Weekly* Flynn announced wryly: 'At the outset we had a definite objective, viz., to investigate the difficulties of wireless in the bush. Humbly we may claim to have attained that objective!'[2]

Radio communication was still an intractable problem. The experimental equipment had proved cumbersome, complex, expensive and not entirely reliable – wholly unsuitable for the needs of the people it was designed to serve. But Flynn refused to be totally pessimistic.

'Amid the disappointments,' he said, 'we were able to point to morse messages safely put over the air from Beltana, Innamincka, Cordillo Downs, and Birdsville; all from gear (8AC) hastily assembled (some beautiful, some junk) and set up temporarily by the wayside as we travelled. Our day of triumph was at Oodnadatta, when we learned (a month after the event) that our speech through wireless telephone from Cordillo Downs station (80 miles north of Innamincka) had been successfully picked up by Mr Hall – a visitor with a roughly made receiving set at Murnpeowie, about 300 miles by air.' However, the main fact had been established – that 'no one with a car (with a bank behind) need be dumb in the bush'.[3] Given that most people in the bush did not have a motor vehicle for power generation, nor extensive financial resources, it was not a huge win. But it was a start. And it gave Flynn the confidence to believe that greater progress would be achieved in the future.

Back in Melbourne after the completion of the hospital at Alice Springs, and with the McKay bequest breathing new life into the aerial services idea, Flynn once again turned his attention to the issue of wireless communication. He planned to return to Alice Springs, armed with an extension on his wireless permit, and continue the search for an ideal transmitting set for bush use that was independent of a power supply from a motor vehicle. To be consistent, voice transmission required more sophisticated and powerful sets than Flynn and his team were able to produce, so reluctantly giving up on that idea for the present, Flynn settled on ICW (interrupted continuous wave) transmitters capable of morse signals only and powered by 6-volt batteries. The idea was to install these transmitters at a number of outback locations within range of one base station, Alice Springs for the purpose of the exercise, which would be equipped with a fairly powerful phone set. Under this system outward messages would be sent by voice and inward messages received in morse. This would at least enable the base station operator to 'play back' the message to ensure that there had been no errors in the morse transmission.

Success of the plan would be dependent on the willingness of people in the outback to learn morse and Flynn was aware of the difficulties inherent in trying to sell that idea. Michael Page, in *The Flying Doctor Story 1928–1978*, makes the point that an operator needed about '200 hours of regular tedious practice to achieve a sending and receiving speed of twenty words a minute in morse code'.[4] Although the Inlanders, in order to send a simple SOS, would not need that level of expertise, they would still have to commit to some sort of training program. Flynn intended to work at persuading the women of the outback households who were more likely to be at home while the men were out on the run – mustering, droving or fencing. It would not be easy. However, Flynn hoped that the benefits that would accrue from the ability to send for help or relay messages of a more prosaic nature – orders for supplies and so on – would reconcile users to the necessary period of tuition.

Needing the help of a specialist technician, Flynn once again contacted Alfred Traeger. Traeger was keen to be involved and henceforth was employed as the AIM's radio expert and electrician. Even as a child the remarkable Alfred Traeger had shown an interest in electronics. He was born in Glenlee, Victoria, in 1895 of German Lutheran stock and grew up on a wheat farm at Balaklava in South Australia. The story is often told of how at age twelve, to the amazement of his family, he had rigged up his own telephone receiver-transmitter with a line running between the family farmhouse and an implement shed 50 metres away. The precursor to the transceiver? Traeger's obsession developed and his father, realising that the boy would never be a farmer, enrolled him in a four-year course in mechanical and electrical engineering at the Adelaide School of Mines. Farming's loss was to be electrical engineering's gain. After graduation Traeger had a number of different jobs and was working for Hannan Brothers in Adelaide when Flynn first met him. According to Fred McKay in *Traeger: The Pedal Radio Man*, Traeger looked like 'a working hand from a wheat farm – unconcerned about social life, content with his daily work, unpretentious, of very shy disposition, and virtually unknown'[5]. Unknown at this point certainly but destined to become, at least in the outback, a household name.

The two men, Presbyterian minister and Lutheran radio ham, who were to become life-long companions and colleagues, travelled to Alice Springs and set up their base in the basement of the nursing home. It was the first of many trips they made together in the pursuit of the illusive radio dream. Traeger installed a 32-volt lighting plant to power the 'mother' base station which had been gifted from Ernest Fisk of AWA. After various tests, Harry Kauper in Adelaide was able to report that he had received both voice and gramophone music from their end. 8AB was on the air. Leaving the base station in the hands of the local telegraph operator, they hastened to Hermannsburg Lutheran Mission, 130 kilometres west of Alice Springs, and set up a crude 'field' transmitter (8AD) and a 9-metre aerial. Pastor Frederick Albrecht and Albert Heinrich, the mission school teacher struggled manfully to master the rudiments of morse code and to learn to operate the equipment. After a few false starts they were able to successfully transmit a message back to base – 8AD calling 8AB – to the jubilation of everyone listening in.

Buoyed by this small victory, Flynn and Traeger departed for the police station at Arltunga, 113 kilometres east and set up a similar installation – 8AE. Before long they had the threefold operation working to plan although the time of day dictated the effectiveness of the transmission. Evening was good and early morning even more so. Successful early morning tests were also conducted directly between 8AD and 8AE. Flynn could boast that he now had a completely self-contained transmitter and receiver, working over 242 kilometres each morning, and costing well under £100. For want of a permanent base operator, this little radio network, consisting of a base telephony station and two outpost telegraphy stations had a brief life, albeit an eventful one, but it formed one more link in the chain of events that would lead to a permanent voice for the bush. They had proved, at least in principle, that radio contact could be made between a base station and a network of smaller stations.

The vision grew. Flynn imagined a 'sprinkling of "mother" stations, each in charge of some good-natured person, generally honorary, able to send out telephone messages and news, or advice, at certain times of the day (mostly early and late), and all around each a medley of "Baby" stations – squeaking out brief questions and thanks for replies in morse.'[6]

This series of experiments progressed the program, proving that non-technical people could be taught to use the wireless transmitting and receiving equipment and to master morse code. But Traeger was not yet satisfied. The gear was still clumsy and comparatively expensive in packing, freight and maintenance. He needed to devise a self-contained transceiver (transmitter and receiver) and a simple type of generator, driven by manpower, which would obviate the unsatisfactory and expensive battery system. Flynn was still confident: 'We think it can be done, but it will be hard to do; just how it is to be done is not yet quite clear, but we are continuing to feel for the way'.[7] They might have to make pace slowly but that was the Inland way. Traeger returned to his workshop and began again – modifying, inventing, improving.

Traeger's next step was to create a hand-cranked generator to replace the cumbersome batteries. It was a cheap and durable solution which provided sufficient power but required two operators – one to work the generator, and another to transmit the morse code message. This process would serve for the moment but would not be practicable in the field where only one person might be present when an emergency message had to be sent. There was also the difficulty of hand-cranking at a speed steady enough to avoid causing variations in the current. Harry Kauper suggested the addition of a quartz crystal to the circuit which had the effect of increasing the stability of the signal even when the generator was driven unevenly. They also modified their mobile transmitter so that it could be operated in the field without having to jack up the wheel of the Dodge. Much encouraged, Flynn and Traeger then set out for Cloncurry to lay the groundwork for the trial of the Flying Doctor Service. A spectacular radio demonstration was staged here for Melbourne Cup Day 1927 in the backyard of the Post Office Hotel. Traeger rigged up his powerful receiver and the townsfolk had the pleasure of listening to the local favourite come home at Flemington. As a means of getting the attention of the locals it worked a treat. The populace was now very focused on this new technology and more than ready to hear Flynn's address in the Shire Hall where he outlined the plans for the forthcoming aerial medical experiment, described the recent success of the radio tests and promised that before long Cloncurry and its surrounding community would soon be linked by wireless. The culmination of the evening came when Flynn invited the deputy chairman of the Shire Council to say a few words to Harry Kauper in Adelaide using the shortwave telephony set in the Dodge. Initially diffident, the deputy chairman soon found his voice, and according to W Scott McPheat in *John Flynn: Apostle to the Inland*, was still talking twenty minutes later![8]

In May of the following year, the aerial medical service made its first flight, and although there was a reasonably efficient bush transmitter now available, it was still not yet suitable to be mass-produced and installed at multiple outposts. The possibility of using carrier pigeons to carry urgent messages, though mooted by George Simpson, never took wings.[9] So the service relied initially on telegraph, telephone and hand-delivered messages for communication between outposts and the flying doctor at Cloncurry. It was not ideal and sometimes meant a flight was made that would have been unnecessary had the doctor been able to communicate directly to the originator of the message. Nonetheless, the system worked well enough for the value of the experimental year to be beyond question.

9

Pedal Power

. . . .

Traeger, meanwhile, was still hard at work. He improved the receiver and made it capable of receiving broadcast programs when the aerial coil was changed. This required the use of earphones but a loudspeaker sufficed when conditions were favourable. But Traeger was still dissatisfied with his hand-wound generator. He agonised over the awkwardness of operators having to use one hand to turn the handle while the other hand grappled with the morse code message. Then he had the idea that would secure for all time his place in the pantheon of significant AMS contributors. Using a principle established by German soldiers in the trenches of the First World War, he devised a generator using bicycle pedals. The operator would pedal to provide power leaving their hands free to send morse code.

The famous pedal radio (described by Flynn as a 'marvel of efficiency') made its debut and became one of the cornerstones of the triple alliance of aviation, medicine and radio. Traeger triumphantly notified Flynn that he had solved the problem of power supply and Flynn rushed to Adelaide to view this new wonder for himself, taking the now-famous photo of Traeger, in his best suit, riding to glory on the pedals of his new invention. Several months later Flynn was able to leave on his overseas trip secure in the knowledge that the radio network was almost a fait accompli. From the vantage point of the technologically advanced twenty-first century, the pedal radio may seem like a very simple device. But in 1928, its development was an enormous breakthrough and one that encouraged Flynn to believe that the solution to the communication problem in the outback was at last within their grasp. As the photograph illustrates, the equipment was enclosed in a metal housing, filled with oil to minimise wear, with the pedals on the outside to drive the generator. The cast base could be firmly screwed to the floor beneath a table on which sat the transceiver contained in a sturdy wooden box. The complete equipment cost £33, a small price for what, in effect, was to spell the end to isolation for the Inlanders. Lonely homesteads and settlements, remote mission and police stations, Aboriginal communities – every inhabitant of the outback would benefit.

With the baby sets in hand, it was now time for Traeger to turn his attention to the mother station that would service the AMS at Cloncurry. This base radio station was set up in April 1929 by Traeger and Harry Kinzbrunner who had been engaged as the base operator. The base transmitter was engine-driven, giving sufficient power for Kinzbrunner to speak to the pedal transceivers (the baby sets) by radiophone once they were in position. Vocal transmission was imperative for the base stations as a doctor's diagnosis and instructions would be too complicated to be trusted to morse. Morse, however, was how the base station would receive the answering messages. This system later sorely tried the patience of the base operators who had to cope with deciphering morse code dots and dashes received from outstation amateurs often transmitting with more enthusiasm than accuracy. Sometimes the messages had to be transmitted and retransmitted before the base operator was satisfied that he had the complete picture. In this way the base operators became legends in their own right, not only for their technical expertise, but also for the invaluable local knowledge they amassed throughout their years of service, which they passed on to doctors and pilots.

The base station had its official opening in June in the presence of three hundred admiring onlookers. Flynn was there in spirit only as he was then on his long-awaited overseas trip. The opening address was given by the chairman of the Shire Council whose praise for the organisation and its auxiliary services was fulsome:

> Just to illustrate the general utility of the service, it might be
> mentioned that the PMG's Department has given permission to
> the AIM Wireless Service to receive telegrams from isolated
> places, and then to be further transmitted by telegraph from the
> nearest Post Office, so you may imagine the blessing that this
> will be to those people so terribly isolated as they are at present.
> Living hundreds of miles from any telegraphic facilities it will
> be realised what a wonderful convenience it means to them.
> This service in the matter of despatch of telegrams, so far as the
> AMS is concerned, is purely a courtesy service and the only
> charge involved will be the regular charge for the telegram by
> the Postal Department.[1]

The capacity of the radio network to transmit telegrams to and from remote locations was an enormous boon and for this role the infant AMS later received much-needed revenue from the Postmaster General's Department (PMG). The PMG further assisted by waiving the conditions of the *Wireless Telegraphy Act* to allow the outposts to be operated by non-licensed people. Ernest Fisk, having already donated much equipment to the AMS, again came to the service's aid when his company, AWA, agreed to make its patent rights available free of charge on the proviso that proposed wireless sets manufactured by the AIM were supplied to outback people at cost price.[2] These concessions were indicative of the high regard in which the service was held, both by the public and by governments.

But first the baby sets had to be installed. Six locations were chosen covering an area of about 233 000 square kilometres. It was important that this be done before the 'wet' set in and made the roads in the north impassable. Travelling with George Scott, the AIM patrol padre for the area, Traeger set off for the first outpost at Augusta Downs station, 290 kilometres north of Cloncurry. Not only did Traeger have to install and test the pedal radio and raise the aerial, he also had to teach morse to the wife of the station manager, Mrs Rothery, and familiarise her with the intricacies of running the apparatus. Learning to work the pedals rhythmically while tapping the morse keys and fiddling with the controls was not easy. Mrs Rothery came through and tapped a tentative message back to the base at Cloncurry. The initial link was established. Several days later the first radio telegram was received at the AIM office in Sydney from Augustus Downs and read as follows: 'Greetings by wireless service from Augustus Downs, first station installed. Manager and family and station deeply appreciate service rendered.'[3]

Fred McKay, in *Traeger: The Pedal Radio Man*, recorded the reminiscences of the event from Mrs Rothery, then aged ninety-two: 'Mr Traeger was a marvellous man and I will never forget his patience. I was his first pupil and I knew he was shy about ladies. But he was so patient and helpful, and he stayed with us about seven days to make sure that I understood everything. He worked quietly and you would never think he was so clever.'[4]

With the first stage successfully completed, Traeger and Scott hurried on to Lorraine and then to Gregory Downs to install the second and third units. The installation of each set proved fascinating for the locals as Padre Scott observed: '[At Gregory Downs] all was bustle and excitement, as a picnic race meeting was to start next day, and the station was thronged with visitors from Burketown, Camooweal, and the surrounding country. About 200 people assembled. Mr Traeger had a very busy time installing the station, which was an object of interest to many who had never before seen a wireless transmitting plant.'[5]

The fourth set was destined for the nursing home at Birdsville where the nursing sisters had been eagerly learning morse code in anticipation of the event. Birdsville, one of the most isolated towns in the outback, 483 kilometres to the nearest railway, 322 kilometres to the nearest telegraph, where it was said that visitors wiring of their impending arrival brought the telegram with them, had at last joined the rest of Australia. Traeger's assignment was completed with a fifth set at the Aboriginal mission on Mornington Island in the Gulf of Carpentaria and a sixth at Corinda.

The missionary at Mornington Island, Rev. R Wilson, described graphically how effective the pedal radio system had been in breaking down their feeling of isolation from the rest of the world:

> Our only link with the mainland was formerly by means of our Mission boat, the *Morning Star*. She brings our mails and supplies, and we have had to wait for a period as long as four months for news of the outside world. Formerly, if we had to send off a telegram, it meant that our boat had to make a trip of 200 miles to Burketown and back in order to lodge the wire and receive a reply. Since the installation of the transmitting set we are able to send our telegraph message from our own home. At a set time every day we are called by the Mother Station, and our messages are sent in morse Code and handed in to the post office at Cloncurry and despatched over the land wires in the usual way. The reply is given to us by voice from Cloncurry next day.[6]

On a radio 3AR broadcast in 1929 Dr George Simpson explained the system employed by the mother station and the scattering of baby stations:

> One expert is always on the mother station at Cloncurry. Each new station has a daily time allotted to him. At this time he listens, and if there is any message, it is sent over by wireless telephony. If the out-station has a message to send, he then gets to work and taps it out in morse. The morse may be imperfect

and slow, but Mother Station has unlimited patience, and anyway
it is the land of wait-a-while. The message is repeated by mother
station by speech until it is all correct. In this way the dumb
Inland has been taught to speak. Isolated stations are no longer
isolated, and the bush is losing that dread loneliness, its birthright.[7]

George Simpson also paid tribute to the painstaking efforts by the
nursing sisters at Birdsville to perform their role as amateur telegraph
operators, a role which must have been far outside the range of duties
they would have envisaged for themselves when they initially took up
their appointments:

> The Birdsville nurses established a record for radio transmission
> recently which will probably never be recorded in the archives
> of radio. Between them they sent an 86 word message to
> Cloncurry to be sent on as a telegram. It took a quarter of an
> hour to send; but pedalling a Baby transmitter is hard work, and
> rests were needed between times. To a real wireless man the
> morse the girls tapped out must have sounded like a message
> from Mars; but Cloncurry got the message, and the Postmaster-
> General a revenue-making telegram. The speed hardly compares
> with beam transmission of 200 words per minute, but it is
> effective, if not showy.[8]

There were a few mechanical hiccups in the operation of the radio
sets which Traeger identified when he was installing and overhauling
the first of them. Traeger himself gave an interesting assessment of the
situation.

> We have found that there is no difficulty for the operators to
> master the sending of the morse code … The difficulty is in the
> working of the apparatus. However from the data gained during
> the present year, the sets can be so designed as to reduce the

possibility of breakdowns by at least 80 per cent. Many unforseen contingencies have arisen, such as danger from flying foxes. These evidently do not see the small guy wires [supporting the aerial] at night, and although the guy wires do not break, they are stretched considerably and become loose, when there is grave danger of the poles collapsing. This difficulty can be overcome by using much stronger guy wire at these locations. Dust has been a serious trouble, and the vital parts of the apparatus will have to be made airtight, as this is the only means to keep the North Queensland dust out. Warping of the wooden cases due to the very severe heat is also a cause of some of the troubles, as this shifts the position of the components inside the case. It has also been found that a two-valve receiver gives insufficient volume for comfortable working, and it will be necessary to add an extra amplifying stage. To overcome this difficulty the sets should be enclosed in metal cases, a duplicate transmitter installed and an amplifying stage added to the receiver.[9]

In his indomitable fashion, Traeger was confident he could iron out these problems. He emphasised the need for a service manual to be published to accompany the small sets, which would describe each part of the apparatus and its function and list likely faults and remedies. He also foreshadowed the desirability of a continual maintenance program so that the sets were not in danger of malfunctioning. This need had been tragically driven home when Sister Gilbert from the Birdsville nursing home became seriously ill and it was decided that an operation in Cloncurry was imperative. The wireless set, which had until then been giving good service, was out of action and, without the means to contact the Flying Doctor, her companion sister was forced to take her to Cloncurry by slow and rough roads, a distance of 640 kilometres. Although an operation was performed at the hospital, Sister Gilbert died twelve days later. It was another grim reminder of how vulnerable the people of the outback were without a reliable means of calling for medical assistance.

Back in his workshop after repairing the Birdsville set, Traeger redesigned the equipment to make it more efficient and reliable and constructed sheet metal cabinets to replace the wooden versions to conquer the white ant problem. Many years later Traeger smilingly told author Harry Hudson that in order to guarantee the pedal sets could stand up to rough handling he used to 'kick all new models around the backyard, and toss them carelessly into the trucks and lorries, to make sure they were bash-proof before they left [the workshop].'[10] With every modification came the need for more inland excursions to replace existing sets with updated models, and to install sets in locations not yet on the air. Thus began a pattern for Traeger of working in the field in the winter months, gaining knowledge about the peculiarities of local conditions, and then conducting further experimentation back in his workshop in Adelaide in the summer months.

Meanwhile the transceiver had found its place – moved in, made itself at home in a corner of the living room or kitchen, and become part of the family – and Inlanders enjoyed the incalculable benefits of reliable contact with the outside world. Again we hear from Mrs Rothery of Augustus Downs station, who no doubt spoke for many others in similar situations when she wrote in a letter to the AIM in 1929:

> Augustus Downs is absolutely isolated during the wet months.
> The river and creeks make it impossible to get away. The wireless
> is indeed a great boon, and the AIM is to congratulated upon its
> enterprise in installing these sets. I have two tiny children, and I
> know I feel more secure in the knowledge that should I want
> medical attention I can have a doctor at hand within a few hours.
> I am very grateful for this service rendered. The station hands are
> also enthusiastic about the aerial medical service. We live on the
> Leichhardt River, 76 miles from Burketown, and over 200 miles
> from Cloncurry. My nearest neighbours are 40 miles on one side
> and 52 on the other. I am the only white woman on the station.

I was a city girl previous to my marriage, and I thought this an
awful, desolate place when first coming to live here; but I have
adapted myself to the ways and customs of the people, on the
fringe of the Never Never, and rather like the life. Of course
I go away for the very hot months although not so this year.
The wireless is a source of wonder to our boys. Some of them
have lived all their lives in the back blocks and have not even
seen a train. I invited them up to listen in one evening, when the
music was very clear. Their expressions of amazement were very
funny. One chap was sitting hunched up, and I asked him how he
liked it. He said, 'It's very good, missus, but I can only hear it in
the off ear. They aren't playing in the near ear'. He had one
earphone on back to front, and thought it was wonderful when
I adjusted the earphones and his 'near ear' was played into.[11]

John Flynn, with his unerring sensitivity to the needs of others,
had precisely pinpointed what was needed to enrich the lives of
Inlanders, and in utilising the genius of Alfred Traeger, had been able
to make it happen.

From the point at which the AIM's group of nurses, patrol padres,
flying doctors and radio experts began their life-saving work,
magazines like *The NSW Messenger*, *The Presbyterian Messenger*, *The
Flying Doctor* and *Frontier News* faithfully chronicled the achievements
of these outback heroes. The tone of these stories became particularly
admiring at the mention of each new development in the radio network. Each additional pedal radio installed prompted an outpouring
about the marvels of this very advanced, for its time, technology. The
following, with its triumphant heading and effusive prose, is indicative:

Innamincka Tunes In!
Like a flash, a radio pierced the silence of the inland, as
Innamincka hailed Cloncurry for the first time. It all happened
with the visit of the Gulf Patrol party, including Padre and Mrs

Scott, Dr A J May (the late Flying Doctor), and the wireless
wizard, Mr Alf Traeger, who installed one of the AIM Baby
Transmitting and Receiving Wireless Sets. From the nursing
home at Innamincka, Sisters Currey and Burchill transmitted the
following morse message: "Having happy time with patrol party;
thanks wireless installation; regards." In less than 30 minutes the
telegram boy appeared at the AIM office in Sydney with the
message. Our wireless assistant at Cloncurry Station had acted as
mediator, picking up the morse from Innamincka, confirmed the
message by telephony (Voice), then relayed it to Sydney through
the local Post Office. Oh, happy days, now that Innamincka
district is in touch with the world![12]

By the end of 1931, Traeger, by replacing existing sets and
installing new ones at fresh locations, could boast that at that point
there were twenty pedal wireless outstations in daily contact with the
mother base. All that was required was for the operator to learn morse
and have some pedalling expertise, more difficult for some than
others. Sister Burchill, despite her delight at having access to a pedal
radio, was one who found mastery difficult and commented self-
deprecatingly, 'I had a special worry about the pedalling. I had never
ridden a bike and could not overcome a tendency to pedal backwards
as well as forwards. Consequently, I lost the cycling job to Ina [her
companion sister] who seemed an expert at it'.[13]

10

The Inland Speaks

. . . .

The Inland, which had initially found its voice via *The Inlander* magazine, now had a much more effective way of making itself heard. The transceiver network became a bulwark against the loneliness and isolation of the bush, exacerbated when flooding cut the stations off from the outside world. Women left alone at a homestead while the men were out on the run could now communicate with the base station if problems arose. The sense of belonging to a wider community was beginning to develop. Broadcast programs were providing some entertainment and the news of the world was finding its way into the most remote outpost. This development was pioneered by Maurice Anderson, the veteran radio operator at Cloncurry who 'listened in daily to the great international broadcasting stations at Arlington in the United States and Rugby in England, and next morning at 7 o'clock would give out the world news throughout the Inland. Fortunate members of his scattered "family" could hear the latest international developments before the city folk read of them in the daily newspapers'.[1] Messages were sent to the mother station and then forwarded to any part of Australia as telegrams, and replies were received on the same day. This contrasted sharply with the situation some years earlier where mail could take months to arrive and news was eagerly sought from passing travellers, a system referred to by the inlanders as the 'mulga wire'. Bruce Plowman, in *The Man from Oodnadatta*, describes a visiting patrol padre involved in just such an exercise. 'As they sat at tea the host and hostess plied the guest with question after question concerning the news of the road and the outside world. Shut off from the road and its travellers, eighty-five miles from the nearest white woman, and three hundred miles from the nearest railway, and with newspapers a fortnight old when they arrived, the good folk were hungry for news.'[2]

So, from being silent, the Inland went to positively shouting. The *Frontier News* of September 1932 proudly listed the amount of traffic in and out of the various bases for the preceding year:

> During 1931 (besides our own traffic for instruction in radio
> and medical advice), radiograms relayed in conjunction with
> Cloncurry Telegraph Office (land lines) were: Outward, 1,805
> messages, representing 39,405 words; Inward, 1,418 messages,
> representing 30,236 words. Our record message consisted of
> 405 words! In addition to the above, the operator at the Base
> communicates each day with the 20 Pedal stations, and many
> consultations are made by this means with the Flying Doctor.
> It is safe to estimate about 11,000 conversations per year under
> this heading.[3]

Traeger's biggest breakthrough yet had come in 1931. Mindful that mastering morse code was a tedious business, Traeger designed a typewriter keyboard to eliminate the need for operators to use morse. It was a clever solution. The keyboard resembled an ordinary typewriter, without the type basket or roller, and was housed in a metal case. For each letter or sign of the morse code there was a corresponding key, attached to a metal arm. On the sides of each arm were cut small depressions. When a key was depressed a roller followed these indentations and registered the relevant alphabetical letter or sign. The message thus transmitted was slow but uniform and required no knowledge of the dots and dashes combinations of morse code. Operators received their message back from the base by voice. Flynn declared the new pedal set an 'ingenious contrivance'. It had been designed so that the average person could use it after an hour's tuition. It was compact, could be carried on a bicycle, had a range of 966 kilometres and cost £70. The new keyboard was hugely popular. Orders came flooding in from people keen to upgrade their systems and be freed from the constraints of morse. It was estimated that this automatic transmission would enable the radio base to handle four times as many outstations as formerly.

At the end of 1932 Traeger went on patrol with Rev. Kingsley Partridge, the patrol padre for Central Australia, with the intention of servicing and upgrading the pedal sets in Partridge's area. The two men began to discuss the possibility of a mobile pedal set that could be carried in the padre's vehicle to enable him to communicate directly to the Cloncurry mother station from the remote parts of his parish. Traeger once again put his inventive powers to work, and by the following year had designed and constructed a compact, mobile, pedal-operated transceiver that could be carried in the field by camel, horse or vehicle. Partridge was the first to use it. The complete equipment was contained in a robust box with the pedals protruding from each side. It was such an invaluable tool that Traeger made a similar unit for the South Australian patrol. Itinerant workers like police officers and mailmen ultimately used these mobile sets also, enabling them to increase the effectiveness of their service to the public.

The usefulness of the mobile set was later endorsed in this account from Birdsville in 1936:

> The Sisters have had a particularly busy period which must be a record for Birdsville. Their last patient was a stockman who had a bad fall from a horse at Mungerannie, South Australia, 180 miles south of Birdsville. The Marree mail lorry passing picked him up

with the intention of bringing him to the hospital here. Seventy-four miles away engine trouble developed and it appeared that no further progress could be made. What did he do? Simply unloaded the pedal transceiver that had been built for his use in such circumstances, and called Cloncurry. The message was repeated on to Birdsville, and in response to his request for medical supplies and spare parts, a car was immediately sent from Birdsville. Under Sister Cooper's care and supervision the patient was transferred to the relief car and had a safe journey to the hospital. This is, by the way, the transceiver's first trip on the mail service, and we all wish the mailman success with his enterprising experiment.[4]

Even many years later, when the telephone system was becoming more widespread, the mobile transceiver still served a useful purpose. Patrol Padre Rev. V Murrell, when stranded at Beltana nursing home in South Australia during a flood wrote: 'The floodwaters were as high as on any previous occasion. Not only road and rail communication was blocked, but the telephone exchange was also at a loose end from the Wednesday night to the Friday afternoon. Here I was able on the transceiver to help various travellers who wished to communicate their whereabouts and safety to their home folk – 8ZD proved itself!'[5]

Notwithstanding the success of the morse keyboard, Traeger was determined to supplant it with voice transmission. He began to devote his energies to telephony and carried out the first successful experiment at Hermannsburg mission in 1933 with Pastor Albrecht in attendance. The significance of this location was not lost on Traeger as it was here that he had installed the first of the experimental receiving sets so many years before. Adding to his satisfaction was the fact that he had developed an enduring friendship with the people of the Lutheran mission during his many radio patrols in the outback, maintaining and upgrading the equipment.

Telephony was an enormously important development. Although the morse keyboard had been a tremendous advance, the Flying

Doctor was aware of the perils inherent in inadequate morse transmission if an emergency required speedy action. How much easier if the outposts could simply speak their message. So it was with immense satisfaction that Traeger was able to announce in 1934 that he would soon be able to supply telephony equipment for every pedal set in the Cloncurry network. By the following year he had achieved that goal. All that was now required was for the caller to pedal the radio and speak into a microphone. Its simplicity made it possible even for children to transmit messages. The morse typewriter found itself superseded. It had been almost a decade since Flynn had reluctantly abandoned the hope of voice transmission due to the lack of expertise at the time. And now, here it was. The Inland had found its voice, literally as well as metaphorically. Flynn was jubilant.

Ernestine Hill, in *Flying Doctor Calling*, commented on the goodwill that the pedal radio engendered and how, as a result, its users were in no mind to abuse it:

> Never yet have I heard a curt reply, nor a fretful complaint of any
> kind, over the pedal-radio – a lesson to the telephones of the
> south. The companionship of the wide air up there is too
> valuable for that. When static is bad, a voice is indistinct, or a
> listener slightly deaf, repetitions are made over and over in
> pleasant intonation, even though the speaker is pedalling for dear
> life with stiff pedals, a dust-storm howling across the iron roofs,
> and the temperature up to 114 degrees.[6]

The radio network had become airborne in 1931 with the first experiments in radio communication between the flying doctor on board the *Victory* and the base station at Cloncurry during a flight. In 1934 Maurice Anderson, the talented Cloncurry radio operator, was instrumental in enabling flying doctor Jock Rossell to conduct the world's first medical consultation from the air. The sisters at the Innamincka nursing hostel had called to report a critically ill woman and Dr Rossell decided on immediate surgical intervention. The plane left at first light and as they flew to Innamincka, Rossell was able to advise the sisters on treatment, while Anderson, battling air sickness all the while, manned the radio. The trip was a long one of 1500 kilo-metres with three stops for refuelling – the first time the flying doctor had ever landed in Innamincka. They arrived at dusk and Rossell performed the life-saving operation.

A significant change occurred in outback life after pedal sets were equipped to operate on voice. The famous 'Galah Sessions' were introduced, so named because of the noisy chattering of the pink and grey parrot. After the medical calls and commercial business was transacted, the network would be thrown open so that people could chat. This they did with gusto unless an urgent call for the Flying Doctor cut through and momentarily silenced everyone. A true sense of community began to grow as neighbours, despite being hundreds of miles apart, spoke to one another, exchanged news about family and friends, announced births and deaths, reported weather conditions, talked about the daily activities in the homestead and on the property. While the flying doctor assisted with physical health, the radio net-work contributed to mental health. It was life-saving daily contact which reduced the feeling of isolation and was particularly appreciated by the women. Although these open sessions meant that the minutiae of everyone's lives became public knowledge, this was regarded as a small price to pay when weighed against the benefits.

A curious aside to this situation was that the person to whom the wireless licence was issued was obliged to sign a declaration of secrecy swearing not to divulge any information that came to hand through the telegram traffic. Perhaps the city bureaucrat who devised that stipulation was unfamiliar with the fact that telegrams sent over the Flying Doctor network were listened to by anyone who cared to tune in.

It was not unusual for the AIM nursing sisters to form romantic attachments during their time in the bush. In fact, it was commonly claimed that AIM stood for 'all in for matrimony'! The pedal radio was the means by which these romances could be developed over distances. Maisie McKenzie, in her book *Fred McKay*, tells the story of an enamoured local exchanging tender communications with a nursing sister until they realised that everyone else on the network was following the course of their relationship with interest. From then on they reverted to morse. In the late 1930s Fred McKay also used the pedal radio when he was a young patrol padre in Queensland, separated from the object of his affections. He later confessed:

> The very first official radio message I sent was to a trainee nurse
> at the General Hospital – over 700 kilometres away. [This was to
> Margaret Robertson who later became his wife.] Everybody in
> the bush heard my telegram because in pedal radio country there
> were no secrets. My mates on a cattle station halfway up Cape
> York Peninsula never allowed me to forget the fun they got out
> of listening to that first special communication I sent to the open
> skies. No wonder. My pedal wireless radiogram arrived in
> Brisbane with this romantic message: 'The longest and most
> loving kiss you have ever received is sent by pedal radio from
> a creek bank near Cloncurry'.[7]

Ernestine Hill spoke of the possibilities, both prosaic and creative, that arose from the community sessions:

> The stations talk to each other whenever their wave-length is
> clear by arranging a time. There can even be a general meeting
> over the air to discuss some matter of mutual interest. The doctor
> will give a health talk or his wife or the matron at the base
> hospital a talk for women ... Some of the stations now and
> again have lightened an evening hour for the others with an
> impromptu concert, a long-distance recitation and a sing-song
> to banjo or piano–accordian when the musterers were in, all the

more enjoyable in that everyone knows everyone. It was musical
Dr Woods who tuned a piano at a station two hundred and fifty
miles out on the rim of a salt lake – Mrs Woods, from their home
in Broken Hill, giving him the A.[8]

How immensely satisfying it must have been for Traeger to know
that his inventive power was the instrument by which people of the
outback could now speak to others and be heard themselves. The
importance of this form of communication was recognised by many
philanthropic groups such as the Country Women's Association
(CWA) and Apex clubs who raised money to provide pedal radios for
those who found the cost prohibitive. The Bundaberg branch of the
CWA was responsible for providing the sisters at Birdsville with their
first set.

While Traeger laboured to improve the radio network, the AMS
was undergoing changes in its structure. Flynn had been working to
extend the AMS to other states and had succeeded in 1934 in securing
the state and federal support necessary to transform the organisation
into a national one. Its brief was to set up a number of sections which
would take charge of establishing bases in their own regions. The first
commission given to Traeger by the new national organisation, now
named the Australian Aerial Medical Services (AAMS), was to build
the base radio stations at Port Hedland in the Pilbara region for the
Western Australia Section and at Wyndham in the Kimberley area for
the Victorian Section. He contracted to do this for £1000 for each
base at the end of 1935. Each base rapidly became surrounded by pedal
radio outposts. The first of these was at Warrawagine station, 225
kilometres inland. The wife of the manager of Warrawagine station
described the excitement of the event:

Dr Allan Vickers, who had pioneered the base at Cloncurry,
came west to start the Hedland Base and in 1935 he arrived at
Warrawagine with Alf Traeger, to install the first pedal set in the

Pilbara district. It was astonishing how many of the station hands found they had jobs to do around the homestead before they went on the run that day! First, lengths of galvanised piping to serve as a mast were hoisted, and strongly anchored at set intervals, to withstand strong winds; and from this the wires were brought in and attached to the pedal set. Lots of adjustments had to be made; but next afternoon Alf Traeger sat at the set and, turning the pedals, spoke into the microphone, saying: 'Warrawagine calling Port Hedland.' He repeated this several times and finally said: 'Over to you, Port Hedland'. And then we all held our breaths and listened. Finally came the answer, 'Port Hedland answering Warrawagine, Port Hedland answering Warrawagine. Receiving you loud and clear'. Magic words flooding through the lounge room and what did I do? I cried! Yes, I think that was the most wonderful thing that happened in my life up North. That was a true Pedal Set. You sat on a chair and turned the pedals as if you were riding a bicycle. Indeed the men of the North, when they'd come to Perth, would always say they couldn't talk unless they moved their feet up and down.[9]

The Port Hedland base had only just opened when the crowd assembled for the ceremony were able to see their flying doctor in action. An urgent call came from Warrawagine for Dr Vickers to attend to an injured Aboriginal man who had fallen from a tree and broken his spine. Fellow tribesmen had brought him many kilometres in search of help. Dr Vickers flew to the scene in the *John Flynn* and returned the man for treatment at Port Hedland. In due course he was returned to his home, none the worse for his experience.

Traeger's long association with the AIM ended in 1937 and from then on he became an independent radio contractor specialising in work for the new Flying Doctor organisation. Traeger formed a company to manufacture his transceivers and others took over in the field to install and maintain the equipment. That year was a turning point for Traeger for other reasons too. Over his many years of devoted service to the Inland, Traeger had largely neglected his personal life. He had watched many of his colleagues enter the matrimonial stakes, including Flynn himself who must have hitherto seemed the epitome of the confirmed bachelor, and he decided it was now time that he did likewise. Traeger married, at the age of forty-two, receiving messages of congratulations from radio outposts all over the outback. Subsequently he became the proud father of two daughters. (Sadly he was widowed when the children were quite young, but in later years married again, and a son further enlarged and enriched his family.) Having devoted his youth to caring for other people's families, he had come to family life on his own account relatively late in life, but when he did he found it a rewarding experience.

Throughout the 1930s Traeger's inventiveness continued without abatement, each new development improving on its predecessor. The high point came in 1939 with the introduction of the vibrator unit, a radio set powered by car or truck batteries, which replaced the need for pedal power generation. Traeger had made his own remarkable invention redundant and the era of pedal radio began to draw to a close. The joke that had had currency for years that you could recognise a bushie when you met him in the street because he had to move his feet to be able to talk was to become an old joke. Nonetheless, old hands still affectionately referred to the new type of set as 'the pedal'.

By 1939 there were 150 wireless sets communicating with their various base stations and orders were flooding in for more, particularly for the new vibrator unit. When the Second World War broke out in that year the 'melancholy' news from Prime Minister Robert Menzies that Australia was once again at war was communicated across the outback by Traeger's radio network.

11

The Wireless Network
in Action

. . . .

The bombing of Darwin and other centres in northern Australia early in 1942 focused attention on the possibility that Australia might be invaded. The heads of the armed forces sought out Traeger, now in his mid-forties, for help in providing current information about the location and modes of operation of the Flying Doctor radio network. Lacking a suitable wireless system of their own, the defence forces were keen to use Traeger's extensive network for the war effort. Fred McKay noted the irony of Traeger, excluded from military service in the First World War because of his German ancestry, now being solicited to contribute to Australia's defence plans.[1]

Such was the efficiency of the radio network, according to Major General Michael Jeffery in a 1998 address for the Wireless Institute of Australia, that General MacArthur, commander-in-chief of Allied forces in the south-west Pacific, called Traeger's transceiver 'one of the most useful pieces of equipment for communication purposes over the spaces of continental Australia'. Jeffery continued, 'The people of the inland were the eyes and ears of the defence forces, reporting anything suspicious. They were given silhouettes of enemy aircraft to enable them to report accurately. Transceivers were also used by the army and police and a special clandestine operation using Traeger's transceivers was set up in Arnhem Land to monitor and report on any Japanese troop movements.'[2]

In an article in *The Age* in 1950, the then Minister for Civil Aviation, TW White, said that the part played by the Flying Doctor Service during the war was 'one of the lesser-known stories in Australia's meagre defences of the time'.[3]

Although Traeger designed the transceiver with a multitude of purposes in mind, he must have found it diverting that his apparatus had evolved from a means of calling the flying doctor to forming a contribution to Australia's defence effort. When further raids were made on ports in Australia's north-west, radio equipment was relocated to Halls Creek. Radio expert Fred Ryle, whose name was synonymous with the Wyndham service, was in charge of the operation, and once he had set up again, carried on regardless, although there and elsewhere, communications were subject to some restrictions in the use of frequencies and in information that bases and outstations were allowed to broadcast. The war brought fresh recognition for Traeger and he was awarded an OBE in the New Year Honours List of 1944.

Traeger's contribution to effective communication in the bush continued apace. For situations when the radio base was closed for the day and needed to be alerted to an emergency, Traeger devised a system using a simple tin whistle. A headline in a Perth newspaper – 'They whistle for the doctor' – succinctly described the procedure. It was a V-shaped two-tone whistle which was blown into the microphone through one end, turned over and blown through the other, each end producing the frequencies, high and low, needed to activate the emergency call decoder at the base station. Uneven blowing had the potential to cause problems, but when used correctly, it was a simple, effective device. It was reassuring for users to know that they did not have to wait for a scheduled session before reporting an emergency.

The burgeoning radio network meant that all sections could play a role in coordinating information in times of disaster – floods, violent storms, bushfires – and in search and rescue work. Not only the bases but also the outstations took part in this vital communications work.

People in the outback used their transceiver sets cooperatively. If a message had to travel over long distances, and there was a possibility of static or other interference interrupting the message, it was usual to transmit to the nearest transceiver with instructions to send on the message. Once the outback people had learned to speak, they were not going to be silenced easily. This system worked similarly from the aircraft. Dr Woods from the Broken Hill base reported in *The Flying Doctor* of 1943: 'The plane's radio is working very well, and during the last two trips I managed a two-way contact with the Base at Broken Hill. Sometimes our signals could not be heard at the Base, but were picked up by other pedal set stations on the network, and relayed on to Broken Hill. We have no difficulty hearing the Base. This arrangement works very well and it is satisfactory to be able to order ambulances and notify Broken Hill of our time of arrival etc.'[4]

Another story recounted in *The Flying Doctor* illustrated the utility of the radio network: 'A valuable mare, the property of a station owner, several hundreds of miles from Broken Hill, has been treated over the radio network of the New South Wales Flying Doctor Service. The owner of the mare called the radio base at Broken Hill, and as a result of an exchange of messages with the stock inspector, the horse's malady was diagnosed and treatment prescribed.'[5]

Even the flying doctors were not immune from requests for help with sick animals as this published account indicates: 'A request came from a property near the Queensland border seeking advice about a favourite horse – an unusual kind of patient for the Flying Doctor. He admitted that he was not a veterinary surgeon, but gave what radio advice he could. The horse is reported to be "doing nicely".'[6]

In 1944 Flynn accompanied the Rev. D McTaggart on a 6440-kilometre patrol from Alice Springs into the Kimberleys and back.

Between Halls Creek and Fitzroy Crossing the stations were comparatively close together and Flynn was able to observe at close quarters how communications had improved from when he made his first journeys in that area. He notes with evident satisfaction:

> Through the wireless network everyone knew we were coming and when to expect us. In one case we were delayed a few hours, and the manager of the next station greeted us with 'What's the matter? It's now four o'clock, and you were due through here at half past eight this morning'. You have to run to timetable in this part of the world now! But it's comforting to know that people are checking you through from place to place, and it would be impossible to tell how many travellers have been saved from perishing because others knew when they were overdue.[7]

This is a tradition which survives to this day although the equipment to monitor those on the move is more sophisticated. Travellers in the outback carrying high frequency (HF) radio are welcome to advise the RFDS base of their whereabouts and to check in at various points along their journey to report a safe arrival.

The radio network pioneered by Traeger became more complex during and after the Second World War. Some networks performed multiple medical sessions each day, traffic in and out from telegrams was always on the increase, and patrol padres of the Inland Mission took over the airwaves on Sundays for church services.[8] As more outposts tuned in, the base operators' work increased exponentially, the pressure being relieved when various state sections of the Flying Doctor Service developed additional bases in their own areas and outposts tuned into the new centres. Radio operators, sometimes assisted by their wives, were the unsung heroes, working tirelessly in often trying conditions to keep the network on the air. They became the medium through which medical, social and business radio calls were effected. Like many Flying Doctor personnel, they worked for the love of the job and for the deep commitment they felt to the people they served.

Some of the bases were quite primitive initially, affording sub standard accommodation and requiring long working hours for modest remuneration. Indeed when the Eastern Goldfields Section was established, there was no base station at all. According to Norma King who wrote its history (*Wings Over the Goldfields*), the first AAMS transceiver for the section was installed in the transmitting station of the local radio station whose technician, Arthur Taylor, offered to maintain the set and act as operator in an honorary capacity. Taylor then scheduled the AAMS sessions between the radio station's normal programs.[9] Later a permanent base was established with funds that had been raised locally.

The base operators were indefatigable when it came to assisting people in their networks. Harry Hudson, during an exhaustive trip around Australia interviewing people for his book *Flynn's Flying Doctors*, listened in to base operator Frank Basden, a legendary figure in the outback radio network. Hudson records the painstaking efforts made by Basden to interpret the needs of a 'mystery' caller when carrier waves, heard as a loud hum in the receiver, drowned out the caller's voice:

'I'm getting a carrier wave through from somewhere but no
voice. You can hear me but I can't hear you. Who are you? I'll
read the list of outposts until I come to you. Switch on three
times for yes, and once for no'. He began reading the call signs of
the outposts, and eventually found the one with the fault. 'It may
be the wires leading to the microphone,' he said. He then gave
detailed instructions for repairs, with yes-and-no-code. In about
ten minutes a voice came through: 'Got it, I think!'[10]

Even when the radio network had been in operation for a great many years, the nurses continued to describe its benefits in glowing terms. Sister Campbell wrote from the Fitzroy Crossing nursing home:

The longer I am here the more I realise what a wonderful thing the Flying Doctor Service base station is with its attendant connecting sets. To hear all the voices responding to their call each morning from away over the range to the coast, up as far as Katherine, and down along the river almost to Derby, all receiving and giving messages, getting advice and help when necessary – all interested in each other – just like one big family. City people can have no conception of what Dr Flynn has done for this country.[11]

In the absence of telephones and daily postal services, radiograms sent by the Flying Doctor radio network played a large part in the life of rural areas. A selection from the archives at the Broken Hill base illustrates the range of issues that were covered – a miscellany of business, domestic and personal matters which afford a fascinating glimpse into bush people's daily lives.

ANY POSSIBILITY SENDING 15 RAMS TRANSPORT FRIDAY PLEASE PAY PARTICULAR ATTENTION TAIL WRINKLES.

WITH RAMS ONE PINT RED HIGH GLOSS PAINT.

FINISHED SHEARING PM 14TH AT LAST STOP 13385 SHEEP 405 BALES AVERAGE WEIGHT 360LBS STOP LAST BALES TO GO THIS WEEKEND PER CULLEN STOP NO LUCK WITH HOUSEKEEPER YET.

WITH ORDER PLEASE ONE SLOTTED SPOON ONE EGG SLICE TWO POSTHOLE SHOVEL HANDLES.

HOPELESSLY BOGGED TICKALARA ROAD WILL ADVISE LATER.

SORRY NOW UNABLE TO BE BEST MAN AS EXPECTING FLOOD.[12]

When telephones eventually took over as the principal means of communication, many outback people, while relishing the new privacy, missed the sense of community that the galah sessions had made possible and were regretful that the highs and lows of daily life could no longer be shared. A poignant letter from Meekatharra in Western Australia, published in the *Frontier News* in 1989, illustrates:

> I wonder about the elderly mother of one woman. I miss the letter of the distant daughter of another woman. She did so enjoy sharing her daughter's travels with others. What about that special little girl, now a teenager whom the whole community loves and cares about? We all rejoiced at her progress. And how are all the ex-School of the Air children doing, now they are away at boarding school or making their respective ways in chosen fields? In town today I saw a neighbour pushing a pram containing a delightful three month old baby! In the past I would have shared in the anticipation of his coming and the joy of his birth. Today was the first I knew of his arrival.[13]

Gary Oldman, a base IT manager who began his career as a radio operator, described the open sessions and endorsed the sense of regret that accompanied their termination:

> The station people knew that everyone was listening in so were mindful of that and were careful what they said. But it was just the accepted way of day-to-day life and they were very good at it. I can remember one property where there was a lady called Mrs Newland who had throat cancer. And when she had to send a telegram, I found it very very difficult to understand. The ladies in the area were aware of this and they knew that not only me but the other operators also had trouble so they would listen in and help. I would ask, "Did anyone get that voice?" And one of the locals would pick it up and say, "She said such and such". Mrs Newland understood and she wasn't embarrassed about it because she knew that she had help. And this really highlighted the flavour of the bush and the camaraderie that existed. It was a shame when that ended.

It was the Flying Doctor radio network which became the facilitator for the famous School of the Air which began in 1951 in Alice Springs and quickly spread to other states. Adelaide Miethke, who had earlier assisted in the establishment of the Flying Doctor base in Alice Springs, once more made a vital contribution to the welfare of Inlanders. She recognised in the radio network a potential teaching aid whereby children of station families could participate in lessons conducted over the airwaves. Educationalists were enthusiastic about the proposal seeing it as an imaginative but practical way for outback children to receive oral instruction from trained teachers to augment their more passive correspondence work. It had the additional benefit of enabling isolated children to interact with others their own age and to learn valuable social skills. Such was its success that this new system of learning rapidly spread to other states. High frequency radio is still an important tool in providing lessons to students in remote areas but in recent years, as communications technology has improved, students and their teachers have also been able to access other media like phones, faxes, video and computers.

A major alteration to the wireless network came in the 1970s when all outpost radio stations were obliged to convert from double to single sideband mode of transmission in line with a worldwide scheme to relieve the congestion in the short-wave bands. The new system of transmission promised to be more reliable and efficient and less susceptible to static interference. It incorporated an emergency call system that was more elaborate than the Traeger system then in operation. It allowed for a signal to be transmitted to the outpost indicating that the emergency call had been received and for a bell to be operated in the control unit at the residence of the doctor on duty who would answer the call and speak directly to the calling outpost.[14]

A coordinated plan was adopted whereby the existing double sideband system would be gradually phased out. The Flying Doctor Service was faced with the enormous and expensive task of re-equipping its twelve base stations, as well as its thousands of outpost transceivers. Traeger's factory lacked the resources to undertake such an extensive operation and in 1974 it was closed down. Traeger's final offering to the AIM was to build single sideband sets for all the AIM field staff, the first one going to the sisters at Birdsville.

When Traeger died at the age of eighty-six in 1980 he had built more than 3000 radio sets for the outback. His sets spread across two-thirds of the Australian continent, covering more than five million square kilometres, a territory as large as Western Europe or almost two-thirds the size of the United States. Many people were involved in the development of the radio network, particularly the base operators, who were like friends to the outback people and gained a special place in their affections. But it is Alfred Traeger whose name is best remembered. Beloved of the Inlanders, his kindness, tenacity and cleverness were the characteristics which brought about this revolution in outback communication. Without this communication revolution the Flying Doctor Service would have been severely compromised during its early operation.

In the years since Alfred Traeger developed the first pedal transceivers, telecommunications and satellite systems have developed rapidly, with telephones now largely superseding radio communication. Whereas a few years ago, all calls for medical assistance were received by radio, today this represents only about 2 per cent of all such calls. People who still rely on the RFDS HF radio network include small communities who cannot connect to the standard telephone, mobile users including exploration camps, Aboriginal outstations and tourists.

Travellers in remote areas are encouraged to carry satellite phones or HF radios configured to the relevant Flying Doctor frequencies in case of emergencies. Flying Doctor bases supply information about what communications equipment is available. When an emergency call is received at a Flying Doctor base, a doctor, nurse and pilot can be airborne within forty-five minutes. Though the nature of the communication system has changed dramatically over the years, it still continues to be a vital link between the Flying Doctor Service and the person requiring medical assistance and advice.[15]

Chief Medical Officer Dr Anne Wakatama says that as rural populations have declined and there are fewer workers employed, certain sorts of injuries have decreased, for instance, those that might have occurred on properties, such as falls from horses or bikes or mishaps with vehicles, tools or machinery. Conversely there has been an increase in other types of accidents because there are more and more people exploring the outback. A growing part of the work of the RFDS is attending these people when they have road accidents, even though they might come from cities way outside the usual catchment area of the flying doctor base. City people thus find themselves in the unexpected position of being recipients of Flying Doctor care when their usual perception of the Flying Doctor Service, if they have one at all, is that it exists to service rural communities. Many of these travellers lack experience in the particular problems of outback travel. For instance, travelling on unsealed roads can offer an exciting adventure but is a trap for the unwary. For the first time the motorist may have to contend with cornering on dirt roads, overtaking road trains, dust that obscures vision, flooded bridges and causeways, or hidden dangers such as holes and ruts. A further pitfall for the uninitiated is the presence of stock and wildlife suddenly materialising out of nowhere.

Gary Oldman concurs:

> There's a lot of inexperienced people who go outback and they're not used to driving in the bush – some are overwhelmed by the distances when they actually do get there. Some can get quite terrified when they're out in the remoteness and there's no one to call on and they're waiting for a car to come along. So satellite is one option even if it's only a straight UHF CB because the bush people use those and there's every chance you might be able to get on to a property for help. An experienced

four-wheel driver who's going bush will at least have a UHF
and either an RFDS radio or a satellite phone – it's just so much
easier. I used to say to people, 'It's not so much for your safety
but you might come across someone who needs your help'.
And at least you've got the means of getting a message out.

The Yulara Medical Centre in the Northern Territory is unique in
that it is the only ground-based facility in the RFDS and the only one
that operates road ambulances. It provides an invaluable around-the-
clock health care service to tourists visiting the area whose numbers
can reach over 400 000 each year. Many come to experience the
climbs and walks on and around Uluru and, in so doing, exceed their
usual level of physical activity. This can result in a visit to the medical
centre for treatment for heat stroke or exhaustion. RFDS staff fulfill
an important role in helping such travellers to recover so that they can
resume their adventure holiday as quickly as possible.

One of the challenges for the RFDS in the twenty-first century is
to remain informed about emerging telemedicine technologies and to
determine how best to incorporate them into the provision of health
services to rural and remote communities. The RFDS has begun the
process by progressively introducing digital cameras and video-
conferencing facilities. When fully developed, these technologies will
enable face-to-face case conferences with other health providers,
visual rather than phone consultation with patients, and speedy advice
and results from specialists and other health professionals.[16]

REACHING FOR THE SKY

12

Aerial Antics

. . . .

In 1928 the AMS began its operation with one pilot, one doctor and one chartered plane flying out of a single base. Communication between outposts and base was by telegraph, by telephone where it existed, or by messenger travelling on horseback or by motor vehicle over inadequate roads. From humble beginnings do great things grow. The RFDS has now developed into the largest, most comprehensive aeromedical organisation in the world. It owns a fleet of 45 aircraft, employs over 500 staff (full time and part time) and operates from 21 bases across Australia. The Queensland Section has bases at Cairns, Townsville, Rockhampton, Mt Isa, Charleville, Brisbane and Bundaberg. The South Eastern Section (formerly the New South Wales Section) operates from bases at Dubbo, Broken Hill, Essendon (Victoria), Bankstown and Launceston (Tasmania). Central Operations (formerly the South Australian Section) has bases at Adelaide, Port Augusta, Yulara and Alice Springs (Northern Territory). RFDS Western Operations (an amalgamation of the Western Australia, Eastern Goldfields and Victorian sections) operates bases at Jandakot, Port Hedland, Meekatharra, Kalgoorlie and Derby.[1]

Throughout the seventy-five year history of the Flying Doctor there has been a gradual increase in the number of bases and in the area they cover. In the last decade alone, eight new bases have been established, the most recent being Bundaberg in 2002, which is operated in conjunction with the Queensland Ambulance Service. As needs have changed over the years a number of bases have also closed down. Carnarvon, begun in 1955, closed in 1996; Geraldton, begun in 1977, closed in 1989; and Wyndham, the second base to be established, closed its doors in 1989 after a lengthy service of fifty-four years. Other significant changes have been in the relocation of two bases. One was Charters Towers, relocated to Cairns in 1972. According to Michael Page in *The Flying Doctor Story 1928–1978*, this was in part a result of the economic development of northern Queensland shifting northwards, such that Charters Towers was no longer in the centre of its 'practice' but at its southern extreme.[2] And Cloncurry, the birth-place of the AMS, was relocated to Mt Isa in 1964. John Flynn Place which houses the Royal Flying Doctor Service Museum now stands in Cloncurry in memory of the town's proud association with the service. There, visitors will find early contributors immortalised in the Fred McKay Art Gallery, the Alfred Traeger Cultural Centre and the Allan Vickers Outdoor Theatre. Gone from Cloncurry perhaps, but not forgotten.

John Flynn worked long and hard over many years to bring the dream of a flying medical service to fruition. At the end of the First World War, when Flynn was championing the use of aircraft, the majority of people in Australia still regarded aeroplanes with some distrust – understandable perhaps, given that many men died in the war flying them. With commercial aviation in its infancy, those pilots who returned from the war unscathed had limited scope to use their flying skills to earn a living. Some became stunt flyers and barnstormed to entertain the crowds. Sir Norman Brearley, who formed Western Australian Airways, the first airline in Australia, suggests in *Australian Aviator* that 'barnstormers were regarded as dare-devil actors who did death-defying stunts in the sky in the same way as wire-walkers or acrobats did challenging feats on a vaudeville stage'.[3] He held the opinion that people flocked to these exhibitions in the hope of seeing a good crash, not good flying!

So while the public thrilled to the sight of planes going through their aerial acrobatics, they were not necessarily inclined to regard them as a serious means of transportation.

Some, however, were more sanguine. The minister in charge of the State Flying School at Richmond, New South Wales, was quoted in *The Inlander* at the end of the First World War:

> I cannot imagine how anyone can fail to see that, as soon as aeroplanes are available, they will not only be commercially useful but necessary as well. The aeroplane has now been brought to such a state of perfection that it is practically as safe as a motor car. The average machine will carry a load amounting to many hundredweights – to tons in the case of big aeroplanes – and its speed places its usefulness beyond dispute. Aviation has become very safe. Information I have received from Great Britain shows that the new machines are almost foolproof. Intelligent men can fly them after instruction in the air aggregating only some 10 hours.[4]

Today's pilots might wish it were that easy!

Aeroplanes were not needed simply because of the huge distances in the Inland. They were needed because, with roads still at a primitive stage, these distances were often not trafficable by any other means – sandhills and flooded tracts of country caused damage to vehicles and delay to anyone intrepid enough to undertake a long trip. George Simpson, on his 7245-kilometre trip around the outback to investigate conditions ahead of the establishment of the aerial medical experiment, listed the damage to his vehicle as a dozen punctures, three broken springs, one broken axle, one broken back wheel and three burnt-out exhaust valves.[5] Breakdowns like these were made additionally grim if the traveller was carrying a summons for help where being delayed could mean the difference between life and death. Flynn chafed at the slow progress in using aircraft to conquer difficult terrain, commenting impatiently in the early 1920s: 'There is nothing to test in aeroplanes. The Q. [Queensland] and N.T. [Northern Territory] Aerial Services Ltd. has gone successfully where boggy roads held up other traffic. Bogs are bogs in that western country – but they don't reach into the air.'[6]

By the end of 1927 Flynn had achieved the seemingly impossible, with all parties agreeing to an aerial medical service experiment to begin the following year. The service began modestly with one DH50 aeroplane chartered from Qantas and built at Longreach under licence from the English aeroplane designers, De Havilland. It was a fabric-covered biplane with an enclosed cabin long enough to carry a stretcher and wide enough for an attendant to sit beside the patient and minister to their needs. It had a cruising speed of 80 miles an hour and a flying range of 250–300 miles, more if a special case demanded it. In addition, the undercarriage had been modified to decrease the chance of bumpiness while landing.

Arthur Affleck was the first pilot for the AMS. His route to that position began in 1923 when he found himself tiring of a clerical job in a suburban bank in Melbourne and began casting around for an alternative career. Rather arbitrarily he decided that becoming a commercial pilot might offer reasonable prospects for the future. He was taken on as a clerk at the RAAF base at Point Cook and six months later successfully applied for selection for training as a Civil Aviation cadet. The Civil Aviation branch of the Defence Department at that time had recognised the need for such training if the burgeoning commercial air services were to be kept supplied with pilots. Two years later he was issued with a commercial licence and after a period with Australian Aerial Services flying their Melbourne to Hay route he joined Qantas in 1927, aged twenty-four.

On 17 May 1928 Arthur Affleck and Dr Kenyon St Vincent Welch, the first flying doctor, embarked on their inaugural medical mission to Julia Creek, 137 kilometres from Cloncurry, and made their way into aviation history books. They were received enthusiastically by the locals at the Julia Creek airstrip, who were well aware that they were witnessing an occasion of great historical moment. In the following weeks the pair made a number of exploratory flights to different centres so that Welch could meet his colleagues and potential patients and Affleck could explore the territory and inspect the emergency landing strips which Qantas had already laid down.

Modern aircraft are now guided by satellite navigation systems that allow pilots to determine their location with great precision. There was no such luxury for Affleck. In the absence of radio and navigational aids, and with only a compass and rudimentary maps to assist, he navigated by familiar landmarks – mountain ranges, rivers, dirt roads, boundary fences and telegraph lines. Eric Donaldson, a pilot who succeeded Affleck, was even forced when unsure of his position to fly low over a station homestead with the engine cut, and yell for directions to the astonished people below. To add to the pilot's discomfort, he flew in an open cockpit behind the doctor's cabin, where he was fully exposed to the elements. Turbulent air conditions, dust, high temperatures and electrical storms made conditions treacherous. Flying was mainly in daylight hours with night flights only attempted in absolute emergencies. And until fuel dumps were established at certain strategic outstations, the danger of these early flights was intensified by extra fuel carried on board in four-gallon tins.

When Qantas first got under way Hudson Fysh had organised for crude landing grounds to be constructed both for routine and emergency landings. He circulated a pamphlet entitled 'A Suitable Landing Ground and How to Receive an Aeroplane'. It gave advice about the placement and dimensions of landing grounds and encouraged homestead owners to send full particulars of their landing ground to the nearest Qantas office. These were included on district maps to be used as guides to pilots landing in cases of 'sickness, accident or urgent business'. So Qantas was already anticipating the use of aviation in a medical capacity. Indeed, a number of such flights were carried out a few years before the aerial medical service was formally established. The final instructions on the pamphlet, entitled 'How to Receive an Aeroplane', show how unfamiliar the public yet were about the workings of aircraft:

> (1) On the approach of the machine a smoke fire should be lit on or near the Landing Ground. This enables the Aviator to judge the direction of the wind, which is necessary for a good landing. (2) See that the Landing Ground is free from stock or any temporary obstruction, and keep people from rushing across in front of the landing machine. Remember the landing speed is at the rate of 40 miles an hour.[7]

In his autobiography *Qantas Rising*, Hudson Fysh illustrates the point with an amusing story concerning a homesteader in far western Queensland, who had never seen an aeroplane before. 'As our plane circled and re-circled his house trying to pick out the most suitable spot to land, he became more and more worried about the failure of the plane to get down. What was wrong with it? Ah … of course! He rushed out into his horse paddock and threw open the gate.'[8]

The landing grounds organised by Qantas, though primitive, were at least a basis for the AMS to build on. Nevertheless, the lack of suitable landing strips and the inadequacy of existing ones continued to plague the Service decades later. The disinclination of homesteaders to create landing strips may have been partly due to the skill of bush pilots who had demonstrated over and over their ability to land in the most unlikely places. In 1943 these problems were outlined in *Flying Doctor*, the journal of the New South Wales Section:

> One of the non-medical difficulties of the New South Wales Flying Service is the need for additional landing grounds for the Doctor's Aerial Ambulance. The ambition of the Service is that

there should be a landing ground at every station in the Doctor's
area, or certainly at every transceiver outpost. Much valuable
work in this direction has been done by many station owners, but
there is still much more to be done. For instance, a few weeks
ago, Dr Woods received a call from a station in Queensland to
treat a woman patient, but the landing ground was short,
although Pilot Bowden was able to land after some trouble.
Before the aerial ambulance could take off, the ground had to
be cleared of another 200 yards of mulga scrub. There was heavy
work in this, and such troubles cause inconvenience and delay.
However, the delay in the instance mentioned had its advantage
for another patient in the neighbourhood. While the plane was
grounded a man came up on horseback, after a ride of five miles,
to say that his wife was on the way to see the Doctor, and would
he wait for her. Dr Woods did, and after treating her, the first
patient was taken in the plane to Broken Hill.[9]

The early pilots were forced to be quite creative in their choice of
places to land and stories are told of landings on claypans, saltpans,
water-logged plains, mudflats, paddocks and sports fields. Affleck
recorded landing on a racecourse track and on another occasion in
the main street of the township of Urandangie. 'The only real hazard',
said Affleck calmly, 'were the telephone lines which crossed the street
from the hotel to Charlie Thomas's store. However, by ducking under
these one could sit down quite comfortably, and having lost speed,
could turn around near the stockyards and taxi back to the pub or to
whichever house one was visiting.'[10]

On one occasion a flying doctor pilot was obliged to land on a golf
course and, after taking off, cleared the trees by such a low margin
that he found gum leaves in the undercarriage.

Today's pilots also carry the burden of difficult landing sites. Pilots
in very remote areas do not consider themselves fully blooded until
they have touched down on a major highway. With more people

travelling than ever before accidents on roads and highways are not uncommon. With this in mind, some roads have been prepared for the purpose. One hundred kilometres north of Glendambo, on the Stuart Highway from Adelaide to Alice Springs, a 1.2-kilometre stretch of road has been widened and a large parking bay constructed to allow RFDS aircraft to land should an emergency occur in this isolated area. The area was built by the South Australian Department of Transport and is known as the 'Traeger Strip' in honour of the inventor of the pedal radio.

There are several stretches on the Eyre Highway also allocated as emergency landing areas. Travellers making their first trip across the Nullarbor note with surprise the presence of these sections of the road which carry signs and pavement markings at either end designating them as RFDS emergency landing strips. Motorists are unlikely though to suddenly find a Flying Doctor plane bearing down on them. In order for these 'strips' to be used the authorities have to first give approval and police or emergency vehicles have to be in attendance to block that section of the road. Because of the huge distances involved in car travel in Western Australia, attending to accidents on major highways is part of the day's work for the RFDS in that state. One such dramatic rescue was carried out by the Kalgoorlie base when a semitrailer, loaded with a cherrypicker, lost its grip and jackknifed across the wet surface of the Eyre Highway. The cherrypicker landed on the cabin of the semitrailer, pinning the occupant under its enormous weight. Once the highway was cleared, the RFDS crew landed and carried out what medical work they could. Then began an agonising wait of eleven hours for a crane to arrive from Norseman, over 500 kilometres away, to remove the cherrypicker and free the driver. By the time the rescue plane had landed at Jandakot airport and the patient had been transferred to a waiting ambulance, twenty-four hours had elapsed. It had been an agonising experience for the patient and a long day of care for the RFDS crew.

It is not only road accidents that the RFDS deals with. In 1999 an accident occurred on the Indian Pacific Railway about 250 kilometres from Kalgoorlie, when a train strayed off its main track into a shunting freight carriage. It was unknown how many people had been injured so flight and medical crews at Meekatharra, Jandakot and Kalgoorlie were all alerted to stand by. Contact was made with the resident nurse at Coonana, 40 kilometres from the scene of the accident. She confirmed that, despite recent heavy rains, the community airstrip was suitable for landing but that it could not accommodate three aircraft. The Coonana nurse advised the medical requirements by HF radio and the Kalgoorlie team were soon airborne. The other two teams departed for standby at Kalgoorlie. When it was ascertained that three planes would not be needed, the Jandakot crew were re-tasked to the south-west region of the state. The Kalgoorlie and Meekatharra crew worked in tandem, and in a well-coordinated exercise, progressively transferred fifteen patients and their families to hospital in Kalgoorlie. The fact that the whole exercise took only seven hours, from the point at which the emergency call was received to the completion of the evacuation, is a tribute to the precision with which the RFDS works. In a finale they could never have expected, the travellers found themselves continuing their journey by train, car and Flying Doctor plane.[11]

There are very strict procedures about landing on a road or highway that does not meet specifications for an airstrip because the potential for an accident is very high. Senior Base Pilot Captain Steve McLay says that one of the problems is that a standard road usually has a camber in the centre to allow water run-off and when a plane is landing at 180 kilometres an hour it can be difficult to hold it in the centre of the road.

Since pilots must land into the wind, determining wind direction is very important. A wind indicator or 'sock' serves the purpose or people on the ground can advise the pilot about conditions. Steve McLay notes, though, that this method can have its drawbacks:

'Aeroplanes can stop at 700 metres, even 600 metres if necessary. At night-time when you're going into unknown strips you usually plan to land and stop shorter than you probably need to – just in case something goes wrong or you get the wrong information. For instance, people say the winds are coming this way, but they're wrong, and you end up coming in with a tail wind that makes you land further down the strip than you intended. So you're always in a state of readiness to expect the unexpected.'

An article in a 1946 edition of *Flying Doctor* outlined some ingenious ways by which pilots gauged the way the wind was blowing. 'Pilots get used to watching certain "pointers". These include cloud shadows, smoke from fires and chimneys, dust raised by wind or sheep or moving vehicles, ripples on water in ground-tanks (the windy side is smooth) and windmills. Birds always land into wind, and animals in a field usually stand with their backs to it. On Monday mornings, or where there is a baby in the house, the clothes line gives the show away.'[12]

13

Landing and Take-off

. . . .

Airstrips are now much more sophisticated than they were when the Service began but some of the difficulties that beset the early aviators still exist, one of which is the presence of animals on the strip. One way around it is for the RFDS pilot to call people at the intended destination on their UHF radio to advise that the plane is approaching. The people on the ground then drive a vehicle up and down the strip at speed to clear away kangaroos or other animals loitering in the landing path – colloquially termed a 'roo run'. So the landing is made safe but when livestock are persistent, the pilot may find the same problem recurring before take-off. Steve McLay elaborates:

> 'There are occasions when you've taxied down and by the time
> you turn around the roos or sheep are back. And you have to
> talk to the station people on the radio and say, "Can you come
> back out here and do another one or two drives and get them
> off". In a drought, particularly, animals come to the edge of the
> strip where there's sometimes a bit of run-off sustaining the last
> of the green feed, and they'll sit there on the edge. As soon as the
> vehicle goes past – they're quite cunning – they'll come straight
> in behind it again and start to chew the grass. And if it's

night-time, by the time you see them, you're already rolling down
the strip and the aircraft's accelerating. You may be past a point
where you can stop in time and you end up hitting one.'

Over the years a number of RFDS aircraft have struck horses or
kangaroos, causing injuries to passengers and in extreme circumstances
the total write-off of the plane. Senior Base Engineer Noel Passlow
tells an interesting story: 'We had a pilot landing at Tibooburra [in
north-west New South Wales] who hit a kangaroo with the nose
wheel on a night flight and the nose wheel collapsed. We ended up
having to replace the nose wheel, repair the fuselage and remove and
replace both engines and propellers. No one was hurt, but the
kangaroo wasn't too good! It just came out of nowhere.'

With advance warning, any other obstacle that has materialised
since the strip was last in use can also be removed. On the odd occasion when there is no spare person available on the ground to inspect
the strip, the pilot will fly low and check that it is clear of animals and
any major ruts. If a call to the station reveals that the strip is not
serviceable, the pilot makes arrangements to fly to another landing
strip close by and those on the ground transport the patient the extra
distance. If the strip is not authorised for night take-off, and the
patient's pre-flight treatment takes longer than anticipated, the pilot is
obliged to take off under Civil Aviation Safety Authority (CASA)
regulations. And again, the patient has to be transported to the nearest
suitable strip. Steve McLay gives an example of such a procedure:

'We once picked up a guy who had been bitten by a king brown
snake in the Flinders Ranges. He had to drive through swollen
creeks to get to a station and the station called us in the middle
of the night. When I rang to make sure the strip was suitable,
given that they'd had recent rain, they said they thought it was.
So I asked, "Can you get someone to four-wheel drive over it and
check it before we take off?" That didn't take long. They rang me

back. They'd bogged the four-wheel drive in the middle of the
strip! That's the importance of getting your information sorted
out. They had to then drive the patient another 100 kilometres to
the south to get to a strip that was higher, in very solid ironstone
country, where you don't get the same bogging problems. They
got him there just as we landed. The doctor and nurse dealt with
him on the strip. Then we flew him out and he was fine.'

Many RFDS destinations have some form of night lighting ranging
from kerosene flares at station homesteads to electric lights at townships that can be turned on from the cockpit with radio frequency. If
all else fails, people on the ground are asked to direct the headlights of
cars, trucks or tractors across the strip to guide the pilot in. Robin
Miller, an RFDS pilot in Western Australia in the 1970s, recounted
the story of coming in to land at Useless Loop (700 kilometres north
of Perth) and discovering an unusual but effective method had been
employed to light the strip. 'Useless Loop itself was well lit by the salt
and gypsum loading installations and the cargo ships tied up along the
wharf, but I had yet to find the strip. I soon caught sight of it, outlined
by two rows of twinkling lights. These, we discovered, were large
powdered milk tins filled with sand and a mixture of petrol and
diesoleum.'[1]

Pilot Captain Peter Brooke says: 'If the pilot thinks he can land
safely on car headlights he'll do it but we'd prefer not to. Numerous
airstrips are classified for daylight only but we also have a large number where we can land at night. Car headlights are a last resort. The
bottom line is safety. If the pilot can do it – fine. If it's a marginal strip
– look at alternatives'.

Some rural communities, aware of the risks to their people if the
Flying Doctor is unable to land, take collective responsibility for the
building of strips or the upgrading of existing ones. Similarly, communities who recognise the limitations of their strip if the Flying Doctor
plane cannot land at night, canvass local authorities or raise funds

themselves to cover the cost of installing night lighting. An example is the town of Baradine, north-west of Coonabarabran in New South Wales. An air space survey indicated that the strip needed extra clearance at each end and on one side to render it suitable for night landing. Using a borrowed bulldozer, people in the town set about rectifying the situation, with the local Forestry Department pitching in to remove the larger trees. The cost of the lighting was supplied by the shire and topped up with local fundraising activities ranging from balls to chook raffles. Their efforts paid off and in the first year of the upgraded strip's operation, over half the landings were at night.

The pilot has the final say about whether or not a flight should go ahead and where it is safe to land or take off. Severe thunderstorms, impenetrable fog or low cloud below the approach levels are problems that cause flight delay, but the safety of the passengers and crew is paramount. If a delay occurs the flying doctor keeps in contact with the patient or carer and gives continuous advice until such time as it is safe to make the evacuation flight or until arrangements can be made to transport the patient to a strip less affected by the prevailing conditions.

In 1928, the first year of the Service's operation, there were occasional disputes between Welch and Affleck about the wisdom of making a flight – with Welch desperate to fly to the aid of a critically ill or injured patient, and Affleck refusing to endanger the aircraft and its occupants by flying in unsuitable conditions. In *Qantas Rising* Hudson Fysh quoted a letter he wrote to Welch which neatly put the situation into perspective: 'It is a pity that Mr Affleck and yourself were not in agreement concerning the state of visibility on the day in question ... We think it is a matter of congratulation that you have a pilot who is prepared to put safety first always. We would like you to think of the consequences to your scheme should the following notice appear – "Aerial Ambulance machine wrecked. Dr St Vincent Welch injured".'[2] Apart from his concern for the welfare of the occupants of the plane, Fysh was no doubt also mindful of the economics of the issue, since aircraft in those days were not insured. And he knew that the damage to the reputation of the Service would be incalculable if any mishap occurred. However, such prudence paid off and there were no accidents in that very important showcase year.

Interestingly, Affleck gives a slightly different version of events in his book *The Wandering Years*, claiming that even though Hudson Fysh had pushed the notion of arriving late but safe, Welch had persisted in his opinion that he, as doctor, should decide where and when they flew. 'Later appointees,' said Affleck pointedly, 'were younger and more tolerant'.[3]

In the first year of operation, with radio communication not yet in place, the number of calls for assistance and consequently the number of flights made was limited. But it was regarded as a satisfactory start. In the following year six radio sets were installed and linked to the Cloncurry base. In subsequent years, as more outposts came on the air and locals became more familiar with what the Service could offer, medical flights increased exponentially as did medical consultations by radio. In the first year of operation of the AMS, 32 000 kilometres were flown from one base. In the year 2002, an astonishing 16.5 million kilometres were flown from twenty-one bases. Although John Flynn had enormous expectations for his aerial medical service, even he would surely never have anticipated that the organisation would one day achieve such a phenomenal reach.

Qantas enjoyed an accident-free association with the Flying Doctor, as Hudson Fysh later observed in his autobiography: 'We never injured a flying doctor or his patient during the whole nineteen years we ran these services before handing over to Trans-Australia Airlines in 1947, rather an achievement considering the type of bush flying involved'.[4]

However, there was one memorable mishap in January 1939 when Dr Jean White, the first woman flying doctor, and pilot Doug Tennant made a forced landing while on a call to the Mitchell River mission in the Gulf area. 'Woman Flying Doctor Missing' declared the *Courier-Mail* at the time, rather ungenerously omitting from the headline any mention of the pilot. They had encountered violent storms after leaving Normanton and were forced to make an emergency landing on a large island in the Mitchell River. Their Tiger Moth flipped on landing and, while neither White nor Tennant was seriously hurt, their wireless gear was damaged so that they could not transmit an SOS. However, the receiving part of the equipment was still operative allowing them to listen in to the messages coming from the search party. They had food and water but were driven frantic by the millions of mosquitoes that infested the tropics during the wet season. In desperation they ripped open all the packages on board the plane and incredibly found two mosquito nets which spared them considerable discomfort. It was four days before they were sighted from the air and another day before a land party could reach them. 'When Captain McMaster circled over the island at 2.35 pm yesterday, both Dr White and Mr Tennant were walking about, apparently uninjured. They waved frantically to him, and he dropped supplies of food and water, as well as blankets and mosquito nets. The nets were probably as welcome as the food, as the mosquitoes in the vicinity are exceptionally fierce.'[5] Little did they know that the stranded pair had already taken care of that particular problem. White was later to pay tribute to the skill of the pilot in landing under such difficult conditions.

Admiration for the difficult role of the pilot was apparent from the first. Notwithstanding their occasional differences of opinion, Dr Welch described the flying expertise of pilot Affleck in glowing terms: 'The more I see of the work of a pilot the greater is my admiration of it. It may be nothing to fly a Moth, but the big 50s are quite different; and to feel one being coaxed out of a deep gully on a hot gusty day, when the air is "thin" and bumpy, would fill you with delight'.[6]

RFDS pilots are among the most capable in the business, given the unusual and difficult circumstances in which they carry out their work. In order to be considered for a job with the RFDS they have to meet certain aviation requirements, designated by the Queensland Section as a minimum of 2000 hours experience as Pilot-in-

Command, 1000 hours as Pilot-in-Command of a multi-engined air-craft and 200 hours night operations as Pilot-in-Command.[7] (When Arthur Affleck got his first job with Australian Aerial Services prior to joining Qantas, his total flying time in command was eighty-seven hours!) RFDS pilots undergo rigorous checks on a regular basis to test their proficiency in dealing with various emergency procedures like engine failure or landing at night with flares. Instrument rating renewals are done yearly and extra engineering courses and flight training are required to qualify a pilot to fly a new aircraft if their section changes planes.

Pilots need to be mature, to use their initiative, and to be capable of working in a multi-discipline environment as part of a team. They have to be prepared to do shift work and this can involve long hours as they are on call twelve hours at a time. Regulations dictate that only eight of those hours can involve actual flying, extending to nine if the plane is already in the air, but this is rare. Pilots have to observe very strict guidelines when carrying out their duties but within that framework they have to be flexible; flight arrangements can change suddenly, flights can be delayed by events out of everyone's control. A pilot on a routine flight carrying an inter-hospital transfer may suddenly be diverted to an urgent case at a bush property or a small community which will take priority. And, along with the rest of the team, they must adapt quickly to the new event. In respect of team-work, Captain Peter Brooke says: 'In the air, as far as the pilots are concerned, from the curtain to the pointy end is their department; from the curtain to the tail is the medical department. In the air they shouldn't interfere with each other but on the ground as far as equipment and patient loading and unloading goes, that's all a joint effort.'

Teamwork has always been a feature of the RFDS operation, not only between pilots and crew but between pilots and the people on the ground. A memorable incident is recounted by George Farwell in *Down Argent Street: The Story of Broken Hill* of the cooperation of people on the ground in getting a pilot to his destination. It concerned pilot Selwyn Woolcock who once made a mercy flight at night from Broken Hill to Bootra (in 1947). In daylight the trip would have been child's play for this bush pilot, but at night none of the usual landmarks were visible. Instead, Woolcock navigated with the aid of lights from homesteads along the way. The radio operator at the base alerted each homestead in turn, and the settlers turned on house lights, car lights and portable searchlights. 'One grazier even offered to set fire to an old shed'.[8] Finally two glowing fires guided him safely to the landing strip.

Early pilots were called upon to perform jobs that extended beyond their assigned role of flying the plane – filling in as anaesthetist or assisting with inoculations. Later there were nerve-racking stories of pilots putting planes on automatic and climbing into the back of the cabin to help out. Norma King, in *Wings Over Goldfields*, tells the story of a doctor taking a pregnant woman to hospital in Kalgoorlie in the 1960s. When the patient went into labour en route, the pilot put the plane on auto and assisted the doctor to deliver a healthy baby girl.[9]

While the main duty of a pilot is to conduct their flights as safely as possible in keeping with CASA requirements, today's pilots also have some informal roles. Pilots help in loading and unloading equipment and in transporting it to the area where it is needed if the strip is at a distance from the medical scene. This needs to be done as quickly as possible as temperatures in summer can make working conditions quite uncomfortable. Pilots also assist when the patient has to be rolled around on the floor or bed to get the mobile stretcher underneath them. Although much of the RFDS work concerns inter-hospital transfers where medical work has already been carried out, there are also emergency situations where patients can be critically injured. In these instances, pilots need a strong stomach to remain unaffected by the sight and smell of blood so that they can walk past the patient, shut off and continue to do their own job which is to operate the aircraft safely. Over time they become familiar with the medical equipment on board and where it is stored so, on request, they can hand items to the doctor, leaving his or her hands free to attend to the patient. Refuelling the aircraft by hand pumping drums of fuel into the tanks where there are no refuelling services, getting the plane in a state of readiness for the next pilot on duty, keeping documentation associated with the flight – these are the range of tasks performed by the Flying Doctor pilot.

14

Airshow

. . . .

All the sections of the Service began their operations using aircraft under charter from various existing air services, for instance, Qantas in Queensland and MacRobertson Miller Airways in Western Australia. The Tasmanian Section began in 1960 with aircraft chartered from local aero clubs, although medical missions (not under the auspices of the RFDS) had been flown in Tasmania since the 1930s. With limited funds available to the different sections as each was established, this was considered the most cost-effective method. It relieved the Service of the expense of building hangars and employing engineers to carry out maintenance and servicing. In addition, the various charter airlines provided pilots as well as replacement aircraft when accident damage or the need for servicing put the usual aircraft out of operation. In the early days many of the pilots employed by the charter companies and later by the sections held engineering certificates. They not only flew the aircraft, but also maintained them.

The first aircraft change for the Service came in 1934 when Qantas replaced *Victory* with a Fox Moth. *Victory* was sold to the Rockhampton Aerial Service, but in December 1935 it unfortunately crashed into the sea off Caloundra, north of Brisbane, while on a regular newspaper run. The pilot survived unhurt and was helped to shore by the Caloundra Lifesaving Club. Notwithstanding its rather ignominious demise, *Victory* still holds a distinguished place in RFDS aircraft history as the Service's very first Flying Doctor plane.

The replacement Fox Moth featured an air-cooled rather than a water-cooled engine and was described by Hudson Fysh as 'smaller, cheaper, easier to get in and out of bad grounds, more reliable, but still single-engined'.[1] A second Fox Moth was based at Normanton for flying doctor Jean White, piloted by Doug Tennant. Their crash-landing in 1939 and another the following year, when the Cloncurry Fox Moth was forced down onto a flooded plain with engine failure, emphasised the need for twin-engined aircraft. A twin-engined DH Dragon, *Dunbar Hooper II*, was already flying from the base at Wyndham in Western Australia under charter from MacRobertson Miller. It had proved its worth by attending a number of urgent medical calls at outposts not previously visited by the Service, some of which it was decided, could not have been safely undertaken in a single-engined plane.[2] Qantas followed suit in 1943 with a twin-engined DH Dragon for the newly established base at Charleville.

The first section to purchase its own plane was New South Wales in 1940. Chartering from ANA had proved increasingly expensive, so the section, despite being financially strapped, took the bold step of acquiring a second-hand Dragon. It was christened *LM Pattinson* after a benefactor who contributed half of the £4000 price tag. Hugh Bond was employed as pilot. And in 1941 Port Hedland purchased the Fox Moth *John Flynn* from MacRobertson Miller, with MacRobertson Miller continuing to carry out its servicing.

Despite these moves, purchase of its own aircraft by the RFDS was gradual, occurring mainly from the 1960s onwards, with each section making their own determinations about when such acquisitions should take place. Initially the choice of aircraft purchased was largely dependent on whatever was available. Later, aircraft were introduced to the fleet to satisfy more specific requirements – increased speed, or greater range or carrying capacity, or night-flying capability. This was in line with the charter of the RFDS to continually adjust its service delivery to better satisfy the needs of its users.

In the 1930s and 1940s aircraft used by the sections were predominantly British – most were De Havilland types like the DH50, the DH83 Fox Moth, the DH84 Dragon, the DH104 Dove and the Australian-built DHA (Marks I, II and III) Drover.

The DH Dragon, and its successor the Dragon Rapide, served various Flying Doctor sections for a number of years. Dr W Scott Kennedy remembers his period of service at Broken Hill in the late 1940s when the Dragons were in use. Although he enjoyed flying, Dr Kennedy admitted to a little discomfort at witnessing the preparation that preceded his first flight with the Service: 'I had a qualm or two when on my first trip I helped wheel VH URE out of the hangar, with its wings folded back along its body, and then assisted the pilot to bring the wings forward and secure them with a quarter inch bolt held in place with what looked like a leather watch band!'[3] A job which Scott Kennedy did not relish but which often fell to his lot was to swing the propeller to start the engines. 'I much preferred to sit in the pilot's seat and look out the window and say "contact" and put up my thumb when all was ready to swing. I can tell you that it was quite a long time before I became blasé enough not to almost fall over backwards after the swing, but I eventually made it and would stroll around the wings and get into the plane, shut the door and seat myself just behind the pilot.'[4]

Then came the Drovers, rugged three-engined monoplanes with features particularly suitable for RFDS work – two stretchers, seating for the doctor and one other passenger, and a wide hinged panel in the door which could be opened to push out food and medical supplies to flood-bound stations and towns. They had a longer range than any aircraft previously used and were fitted with toilets, water tanks, two-way radios, and medicine and instrument cases. In the 1950s the New South Wales Section purchased two, and Queensland operated four under charter from TAA (Trans-Australia Airlines). Their one drawback was that they were underpowered.

By the end of the decade the New South Wales Section had decided that the Drover's length of service could be extended if they were re-engined and De Havilland were asked to submit quotes for the work. It became apparent that the cost of this exercise would be decreased if other aircraft operators could be persuaded to share the engineering costs. The Queensland Section was approached and De Havilland won the contract to re-engine six Drovers, two for New South Wales and four for Queensland, at an average cost of £16,000 per aeroplane. In explaining the rationale behind the move, John Bilton, in *The Royal Flying Doctor Service of Australia*, quoted the President of the New South Wales Section who said in 1959: 'The decision to spend such a large sum of money was not arrived at without a great deal of consideration and advice from leading aviation experts throughout the Commonwealth, including Qantas, TAA and ANA. We were told that there was no plane other than the Drover that was built for Flying Doctor work, and if the Drovers were re-engined, they should prove excellent machines and fly satisfactorily for another ten years'.[5] Weighed against the replacement cost for any comparable aircraft, it was judged a cost-effective arrangement.

Unfortunately, the re-engined Drovers did not fulfil early estimates of their long-term suitability and the New South Wales Section, by the mid-1960s, was beginning to discuss replacements. By 1967 the New South Wales Section had introduced a new aircraft, the Beagle, which served for many years, the downside being that landing strips throughout the network had to be lengthened to accommodate it. In the late 1960s the Queensland Section replaced their obsolete Drovers with Queenairs and once again achieved significant improvements in speed and range.

From the 1950s to the 1970s, American aircraft like the Beechcraft Baron, Travelair, Queenair and Duke, the Cessna 180, 182 and 421B, the Piper Cherokee, Chieftain and Navajo predominated over the earlier British models.

The Western Australia Section, having used a number of different aircraft since its inception and wanting to standardise its fleet, bought a Cessna 180A in 1958 and gradually added three more, two based at Port Hedland, one at Meekatharra and one at Carnarvon. MacRobertson Miller Airways, who had been providing planes at Wyndham and Derby, advised the Victorian Section of its decision to re-equip its fleet with longer-range aircraft, thus eliminating the need for one of its planes to be based at Derby. The section took the step of buying its own plane and in 1959 a twin-engined Dove, *HV McKay*, began service at Derby.

Buying and then upgrading aircraft to suit changing requirements was regarded as paramount by all the sections, although raising the funds to do so continued to pose problems. The Eastern Goldfields Section, conscious of the large sums being expended on charter flights, launched a determined fundraising effort in 1959, and supported by service clubs and other interested parties, raised enough money to make possible the purchase of their first aircraft, a Cessna 182.

However, a few short years later, the section was once again considering a replacement aircraft, one which could cover with greater safety the immense distances involved in many flights in the area. The Federal Council's *Annual Report* of 1962 noted that the West Australian and Eastern Goldfields sections were contemplating replacement of aircraft and expressed the hope that the sections would purchase the same type of aircraft. This was in line with the Service's determination to achieve, where possible, economies of scale in initial purchases and in spare parts holdings.

The two sections complied. Eastern Goldfields chose a twin-engined Beechcraft Baron and Western Australia, which was finding its Cessna aircraft not up to the demands placed on them, followed suit. Dr Harold Dicks went to America in 1963 and returned with a like model, albeit a second-hand version. In describing the reasoning behind the decision to purchase overseas, Michael Page, in *The Flying Doctor Story 1928–1978*, says that the minerals boom had created such a demand for light aircraft that their cost in Australia had become prohibitive.[6]

The minerals boom of the 1960s had additional repercussions. Prospectors, geologists, workers in exploration and mining companies, and their families, swelled the population of the Goldfields area. There were numerous motor vehicle and industrial accidents, increased demand for emergency and clinic flights, and a greater number of outposts making radio contact with the base, all pointing to the need for another aircraft big enough to handle the extra workload. A turbo twin-engined Piper Navajo was acquired in 1969, the first of its type in the RFDS fleet. With a high-speed performance, short take-off and landing requirements, and room for three stretchers or five patients, it ideally suited the needs of the RFDS. Other sections followed this lead and Piper Navajos and Piper Chieftains were the predominant aircraft in the fleets of the Eastern Goldfields, West Australian and South Australian sections in the 1970s and 1980s.

An ongoing problem for the RFDS has been the rapid advance of aviation technology with its built-in obsolescence factor. This has meant that hardly a year has gone by in the last few decades when the Service has not been faced with the onerous financial burden of purchasing new aircraft for one or other of its sections. And with each passing year the cost of replacement aircraft has escalated enormously.

A significant development occurred in 1972 when the West Australian operation became the first in the RFDS to purchase a pressurised plane. *Airdoctor One* was a Beechcraft Duke, bought in America and flown to Australia by Dr Harold Dicks and Robin Miller, the latter describing the plane as 'a joy to fly'. This was a milestone in the history of RFDS aircraft acquisition. Hitherto, in the non-pressurised aircraft, patients with injuries that would be adversely affected by higher altitude flying had to be transported at sea-level pressure, that is, the aircraft had to fly at low altitude so that there was no pressure on the patient other than what there was on the ground. This meant flying through violent turbulence if the weather was unfavourable, a situation which could be agonising for the person with the injury.

Captain David Munns, a long-time pilot with the West Australian operation, commenting on the purchase of the Duke in *The Flying Doctor* (Western Australia Section), said:

> With the introduction of pressurisation we started to see a decrease in morbidity while in flight, especially the very sick premature babies. At last we were able to save these tiny lives. The introduction of pressurisation allowed us to operate a lot higher than we were used to and this put us into a level that permitted more smooth air operations and a smoother ride for the patients. It did not always mean that we were above the weather, but coupled with the weather radar that the Duke was equipped with, we were able to avoid the worst of it.[7]

Despite the obvious advantages of this type of plane, financial constraints prevented the other sections from following this trend. The Federal Council of the RFDS in its 1983 *Annual Report* made the following points: 'Although the Western Australian Section has operated pressurised aircraft for some years, no other Section has followed, mainly due to the high cost of the aircraft. From time to time the Federal Medical Committee has been asked for its opinion on the use of the pressurised aircraft and the answer to date has been "desirable, but not essential"'.[8] However, the medical committee had obviously begun to change its mind and the report goes on to note that the medical committee was now in favour of pressurised aircraft.

Another negative for the pressurised aircraft in the view of the Queensland Section was their small doors which did not accept a patient on a stretcher. However, when the time came for the section to consider replacing its Queenair B80s, the Beechcraft Kingair was well into production and included the fitting of a wide cargo door. Queensland bought a Kingair B200C for its fleet in 1984, the first section to do so, and the aircraft began operating from Cairns.[9] Prior to this development, RFDS aircraft were all piston engined, so the acquisition of the Kingair turbo prop, pressurised and airconditioned, with a higher cruise speed than other aircraft in the Service, was regarded as another milestone in RFDS aviation activity. The slightly smaller Kingair C90s were later added to the Queensland fleet and both types of aircraft were adopted by various other sections.

South Australia was the last of the sections to own an aircraft, making its initial purchase in 1965. In the early 1980s the fleet was comprised of Piper Chieftans and Navajos but later in the decade the section introduced the Kingair B200C to its service. The aircraft was fitted out medically to meet the requirements of retrieval specialists from the major hospitals in Adelaide. An innovative invention – the stretcher-loading device – was conceived during the plane's fitout by an engineer involved in the work. It was designed to lift the patient and stretcher using a forklift principle which spared the flight crew the physical strain of loading the patient themselves.[10] The New South Wales Section also progressively introduced Kingairs to replace their Nomads.

After five decades of operating piston-engined aircraft exclusively, the Western Australia Section acquired its first turbine aircraft in December 1985. The acquisition of the second-hand Cessna Conquest II marked the beginning of a new era in medical aviation for the section. Patients could now be flown from Port Hedland direct to Perth in three hours, a significant improvement on the Piper Navajo which took double the time for the same distance. The introduction of this aircraft, complete with wide door modification, was expected to greatly enhance the standard of comfort and inflight treatment available to patients. The aircraft was medically configured by the section's engineering personnel at Jandakot to accommodate two stretcher patients comfortably with sufficient room for crew and associated items of medical equipment.[11]

These aircraft were vastly different from those used in earlier times, or even in the 1960s and 1970s. The patients and crew were no longer subjected to the constrictions of a cramped, noisy cabin in a slow-speed aircraft flying in the turbulent air conditions which characterised Inland weather patterns. Pressurised, airconditioned, with greater cabin space and an increased range of medical equipment, the Beechcraft Kingair and Cessna Conquest models made life much easier for the working doctors and nurses.

The Beechcraft Kingair, in particular, developed a significant presence in the RFDS fleets and in June 2002 there were twenty-nine B200s in the national fleet. According to the *Australian Council Annual Report 2002*, the B200 is still the 'aircraft of choice' in the Queensland and South-Eastern sections. The RFDS believes that medical services in remote areas should not suffer a poor comparison with those available to urban dwellers. But the desire to achieve better and better standards of service means that the RFDS no sooner upgrades parts of its fleet than improved models become available and the process starts all over again. The newest type of plane to be included in the RFDS fleet is the Pilatus PC12.

The Swiss-made Pilatus PC12 was added to the South Australian fleet in 1995 with the intention that it would eventually replace all the aging Navajo and Chieftain aircraft. It is a revolutionary design, one of the most advanced single-engine turbo prop aeroplanes in the world. It has many features that make it highly suitable for RFDS work – spacious interior, quiet cabin environment, large cargo door and additional forward door, and a hydraulic stretcher-lifting device that ensures an easy loading process. After many years of twin-engine operation the advent of a single-engine aircraft into the RFDS fleet has been the subject of intense study by Central Section and interest by other sections. Queensland and Western Operations have only recently introduced the PC12 into their fleets and operational evaluation of these aircraft is still in progress.

Since the RFDS began purchasing its own aircraft, there have been many different models in operation, but with the current movement towards two tiers of aircraft, B200s and PC12s, the fleet is now more rationalised than at any time in its history.

15

Flying Intensive Care Units

. . . .

Flying Doctor aeromedical planes are not like ordinary aircraft. It takes months of work and around $700 000 to transform a plane like a Kingair into a flying intensive care unit. One side of the aircraft is peeled back and the frame is strengthened to support the weight of a large cargo door. This has to be installed to allow sufficient width for the easy entry of a stretcher. Senior Base Engineer Noel Passlow comments, 'Originally the stretcher had to be physically lifted in through the standard door and rotated to get it into the plane which created some interesting moments for the staff – and the patient. We weren't allowed to tilt the patient through more than about eight degrees.' Noel explains that the normal floor of an aircraft is lower in the middle to allow headroom for passengers but as this does not lend itself to putting stretchers in and out easily, it is replaced with a lightweight flat floor. The aeroplane is fitted with special power outlets for the various pieces of medical equipment and a medical suction system is installed to provide suction for patients who are aspirated. The aircraft requires two oxygen systems – the aviator's oxygen system which is already fitted into the plane – and an additional medical oxygen system separate from that required for pilots and crew. Brackets are also installed for the medical equipment – medical cabinet, equipment poles, stretchers – and the aircraft is fitted with a stretcher lifter. The internal modifications are reversible and it takes around twenty minutes to change an aeromedical aircraft back into a passenger plane.

Because of the nature of their work, RFDS planes land a lot more than conventional planes, making close on 50 000 landings per year over the whole fleet. And they often have to land on soft airstrips. For this reason they are fitted with a high flotation undercarriage where the main wheels are physically bigger than on a normal aircraft and the tyre pressure is lower, allowing a bigger footprint on the tyre. The plane can then land more easily on a sandy or boggy strip.

RFDS planes are fitted out with a full set of equipment for most emergencies except major procedures. These include Propaq units which are hooked up to the patient to monitor blood pressure, heart rate, oxygen saturation, ECG and respiration rate; defibrillators which give an electric shock to restore heart rhythm; ventilation equipment used to keep seriously ill patients breathing; equipment for administering intravenous fluids during flight; gear for delivering babies; cabinets full of instruments and drugs; and vacuum mattresses, vacuum splints and collars for suspected neck fractures. Vacuum mattresses are like beanbags. The patient is laid on them and a pump takes out the air between the beans making it rigid so that the patient can be lifted easily.

With all the equipment on board, the plane resembles a small doctor's surgery or a flying intensive care unit, although there is a limit to what is done on the plane. Chief Medical Officer Dr Anne Wakatama explains that, in general, invasive procedures are carried out prior to flight to stabilise patients so that they can be safely conducted to hospital. These procedures may include the insertion of chest drains or endotracheal tubes to enable the patient to be ventilated.

On the aviation side much prominence is, of course, given to the pilots, even to the aeroplanes themselves which are also players in the drama of RFDS activities. But behind the scenes are the quiet achievers – the engineers – who on a daily basis and throughout the life of the aircraft carry out all the vital checks, tests, inspections, servicing and maintenance events that keep the aircraft airworthy. They are the unsung heroes, out of the spotlight, working to make sure the RFDS maintains its excellent safety record. Noel Passlow explains it in this way: 'The aircraft maintenance side of the RFDS – and I say this without malice, it's just a statement of fact – is fairly much a forgotten thing in all the hype of publicity because we don't exist for people – people don't want to see engineers working on aeroplanes – they want to see doctors and pilots flying into emergencies and saving lives.' However, Noel remembers a time when an engineer *did* take centre stage on a priority one flight. 'A cook at one of the stations near Tibooburra had actually got her hand caught in the mincer and before the medical people could do anything for her, [engineer] Rod McCardell had to go up there and actually cut the mincer off her hand with a friction cutter. It was in one of those big cast iron mincers and she was pushing stuff in and her hand got caught and they couldn't get it out. So that was one of the more interesting incidents that the engineers have got involved in.'

As well as their customary role of taking medical staff to clinics and transferring patients to hospitals, RFDS planes have been used in numerous humanitarian roles like search and rescue missions or dropping supplies and medicines to homesteads isolated by floods. A story from Ruth Deakin illustrates:

> During the years 1948 to 1954 my husband Jack was employed
> by the Western Lands Department to work the dingo fence on
> the New South Wales and Queensland border. We lived at
> Adelaide Gate and our section of the fence extended from
> Bindarra Gate, about sixteen miles east, to Wompah Gate, about
> eighteen miles west of Adelaide Gate. Twice during these years
> the Booloo River in Queensland flooded. When the Booloo

River was in flood it flowed down through the border fence into New South Wales in about eight different places. It was all low lying country so it spread over a wide area. This was called the channel country. It was all broken black ground and when wet was almost impossible to get through even on horseback and, in a vehicle, completely impossible. So at Adelaide Gate we were flooded in on a six-mile island, marooned sometimes for months waiting for the water to recede. In a lighter flood the furthest we could travel was to Teurika Homestead about 14 miles from our home. During a bigger flood we could not even travel that far. At these times our transceiver to the Flying Doctor base at Broken Hill became our lifeline to the outside world. Shortage of food was a problem to be faced when marooned by the floods and it was the Flying Doctor Service that dropped emergency food supplies to tide us over.[1]

Fifty years later the same care and concern is still apparent in this story from Central Operation's magazine *Airdoctor*:

I think the thing that makes the RFDS so marvellous is the personal nature of it. The people of the RFDS really care. I say this from firsthand experience because when my husband Tom's mother became ill, she was flown back home for the last three weeks of her life after a major operation at the Royal Adelaide Hospital. They turned out to be a wonderful three weeks for her. She was near home, but the thing that really made it was the flight to Kingston with the RFDS. You see, when they arrived to pick her up she had just one wish; to see Tom's property one more time. The pilot and the nurse were so kind to her. They flew low over the property on the way in and Tom's mother was just convinced that she had seen some of the cows. The experience meant everything to her. She talked to all of us about the pilot, how handsome he was, and how he'd flown right over the property so she could see the cattle. She seemed to get so well for those three weeks. I think they are a special breed of person at the RFDS; they inspire confidence and still have signs of that pioneering spirit. Hopefully that will never die.[2]

Talk to anyone in the bush and they will tell you about a trip – or trips – that they or a family member or a friend has made with the Flying Doctor. Parents will tell you about occasions when they have sat with a desperately sick or injured child in their arms, willing the Flying Doctor plane to appear, straining to make out the distant hum of aircraft engines. And they speak in emotional terms of the relief when at last they hear that familiar sound and know that the long wait is over. Such an intimate connection with the Service means that users understand its value very well. Contact with the RFDS for bush people covers a full range. It might be a routine visit to the clinics for an antenatal check or an immunisation or to have a sun spot inspected, or a transfer to a city hospital for elective surgery, or an emergency where the availability of the Flying Doctor Service might literally spell the difference between life and death. It is therefore understandable that a great deal of community effort in the bush goes towards raising funds to keep the Flying Doctor in the air.

The RFDS is a not-for-profit charitable organisation and, although it receives funding from the Commonwealth, state and territory governments, it also relies heavily on donations from the general public, small businesses and the corporate sector to help purchase new aircraft and to modify them into flying intensive care units. Due to the low relative value of the Australian dollar, the cost of purchasing each new aircraft has ballooned from $4.5 million to more than $7 million. The cost of fuel and spare parts has similarly increased. So an integral part of the working day of the Service and its army of supporters and volunteers is fundraising, and this has been the case since its very beginning.

The very first fundraising effort could well have been by John Flynn's sister Rosetta who conducted the Ladies' Page in *The*

Messenger, the magazine of the Presbyterian Church of Victoria, under the pseudonym 'Cousin Charlotte'. W Scott McPheat, in *John Flynn: Apostle to the Inland,* gives an account of how this was managed. It was at the time, 1910, when Flynn was keen to amass funds to underwrite an investigative trip to Central Australia and the Northern Territory to report on medical and religious conditions there. Anxious not to be seen as the instigator, Flynn contrived a plan whereby a friend would write to 'Cousin Charlotte' deploring conditions in these remote places and charging readers to offer financial support towards some remedial action. This was the beginning of the imaginative 'quarter-of-a-mile of threepenny pieces campaign' which, inch by inch, raised sufficient funds for the Australian Board of Missions to undertake the investigation.[3] The board appointed Flynn, as had been his private hope, to carry out the survey. As we have seen, this led to the launching of the AIM of which Flynn was the superintendent, then to the development of the network of cottage hospitals, and ultimately to the creation of the AMS. And the rest, quite literally, is history.

Since then, fundraising has turned into an art form and there is no limit to the ingenuity and creativity employed by supporters of the RFDS to keep their Service in the air. At various times and in various states there will be some form of fundraising occurring – outback air races, golf tournaments, walkathons, music festivals, garden open days, art exhibitions, market days, stands at the Royal Easter Show, cycling treks, trail rides, rodeos, gymkhanas, raffles and radio appeals. Auctions for the RFDS range from bulls to a toilet seat painted by artist Pro Hart. Or it might be a tractor drive from Perth to Cloncurry or a golf tournament at Roxby Downs where players tee off, undaunted by heat, flies or dust. If cricket is your game, the MCG (Moomba Cricket Ground), where the Strzelecki and Sturt Stony deserts meet, is the place to see two teams clash for desert cricket's prized crown, the Cooper Cup. The adventurous can try a 'Drop for the Doc' parachute jump at Augusta in south-west Australia and traditionalists can attend the famous Birdsville Races, where for one memorable day each year this outback town's population swells from around ninety to several thousands, as people from all parts of Australia gather to enjoy a day at the races and a great party. They come using various modes of transport and there are often up to three hundred aircraft parked nearby.

Those with a taste for high living can take part in the popular RFDS annual fundraising event, Wilpena Under the Stars – a night of music, fun and fine dining in the stunning outback setting of Wilpena Pound, in the Flinders Ranges National Park, where revellers wine and dine before dancing the night away under a star-filled sky. Similar black tie events are also held in other parts of Australia both in traditional venues and in more unusual locations including woolsheds and aircraft hangars. If your tastes are simpler, get involved in 'operation pudding' and buy a Christmas treat from one of the many RFDS women's auxiliaries.

If you're keen to contribute to one of the biggest fundraisers for the RFDS, try the Outback Car Trek which in 2002 celebrated the Year of the Outback with an epic eleven-day journey from east coast to west coast. The route snaked from Coffs Harbour in New South Wales, north to Winton in Queensland, through the Red Centre and across Western Australia to Perth. The proud objective of the Outback Car Trek over its thirteen-year history has been for participants to have fun, see Australia and raise money for the RFDS. Participants will attest to the first two and, as for the last, the $6.4 million which has been raised since trekking began speaks for itself.

If you want to be amused while you donate to the RFDS there are plenty of opportunities. Tourists on a coach tour in South Australia found themselves subjected to 'sin tin' fines for trifling misdemeanours like calling the coach a 'bus', swearing, heading into the wrong toilets, being the last on board – proceeds to the RFDS. Dog lovers can compete in an ongoing tussle between Western Australia and Victoria to see which state can assemble the longest queue of utes containing a canine – the famous 'dog in a ute' event. Western Australia currently holds the title but a re-match may be pending.

And travellers stopping at roadside stores or cafés in rural areas might encounter a handwritten sign on a cash register bearing the intriguing lettering 'YCWCYODFTRFDSTY'. The inquisitive may be tempted to ask what it means. The reply will be 'Your curiosity will cost you one dollar for the Royal Flying Doctor Service. Thank you'.

CARE FROM THE AIR

16

Sister Myra Blanch

· · · · · · · · · ·

The first nursing sister to be formally employed by the RFDS was Myra Blanch at Broken Hill in 1945. Although her position was termed 'flying sister', she in fact generally used aircraft only for transport. Most of her travelling around the area was by motor vehicle or even on horseback. Indeed, in the job description issued over the Broken Hill network at the time of her appointment, there was no mention at all of her being required to accompany the doctor on emergency or clinic flights. Instead, the first flying sister was expected to engage in home nursing; to relieve nursing staff in emergency cases in hospitals within the area of the Flying Doctor Service; to give advice and help on matters of public health and prevention of disease; to give medical advice when necessary including ante- and postnatal advice; to broadcast talks over the network on subjects of medical interest; to give talks to schools; and to perform medical surveys and immunise children within the area. In addition, it was intended that the flying sister should, in the course of time, visit every homestead within her jurisdiction, particularly those without radio or telephone communications.[1] It was a full program.

The concept of a flying sister had first been raised in 1936 by Adelaide Miethke. As mentioned earlier, Miethke was president of the

Women's Centenary Council. This was an organisation representing over one hundred women's committees in South Australia, which had been formed to raise funds to commemorate the work of South Australian women pioneers. Their idea was to fund a flying sister, based in Port Augusta, to provide health and social services to isolated women in the northern areas of the state. Instead, Flynn persuaded Miethke's group to divert their funds towards the establishment of a Flying Doctor base at Alice Springs, which they did, and the flying sister idea went to ground.

It was resurrected again at a council meeting of the New South Wales Section in August 1944, when a report was presented setting out the advantages and disadvantages of a flying sister. Perhaps the idea emanated from Adelaide Miethke's initial proposal, perhaps not. Either way, a sub-committee later discussed the question, recommended the appointment of Sister Blanch (who was then serving with the Australian Army's Nursing Service), and negotiated with the Manpower Authorities for her release.[2] Before the war, Sister Blanch was in charge of the AIM nursing home at Innamincka. She started her new role in Broken Hill in November 1945.

Sister Blanch took on her tasks with gusto. Reports of her field trips indicate she was a woman with boundless energy, possessed of a very straightforward and authoritative manner. She quickly summed up the medical and living conditions of those she visited and, as the following account suggests, did not pull any punches when it came to suggesting remedial action:

> Returned to Tibooburra in the evening with the police
> constable, thus saving a wait of three days in Milparinka. The trip
> took just one week, and was interesting, profitable, and to me
> enjoyable. My principal impressions were the readiness of the
> people to co-operate in the matter of transport, and the
> regrettable prevalence of what the people concerned just
> described as 'sore eyes' and 'colds'.

The eyes, we are convinced, are definitely infective, and the infection passed from one to the other by flies, also in some cases, by mothers ignorantly using the same face cloths when cleaning the children's faces. Nets, worn right over the face, and tied under the chin, have been freely advocated by the Flying Doctor, and, in most cases, mothers do make an honest attempt to make the children wear them. I have found that when the children do wear the nets, they usually have half the net in their mouths with a dozen or so flies thickly clustered about the nice, moist portion of the net, a very convenient way of spreading germs of summer diarrhoea and dysentery. The summer diarrhoea is epidemic, but conjunctivitis seems to be always with us. I think I know the source of the present trouble – unfortunately, a homestead I was not able to visit.

The chronic cold, we think, is largely a catarrh caused by the continual irritation of mucous membranes by dust, which has been very bad, and always is for a long period during summer.[3]

A staunch supporter of the doctor's view of prevention being better than cure, Sister Blanch was nonetheless aware of the difficulty for some settlers in reporting early signs of illness when they had no means of communication. Her answer was to urge a cooperative approach:

One of the chief problems at present is how to keep in touch with those families which are not on the pedal radio network, and of whom we hear little or nothing until the actual need for assistance has arrived. In one recent instance we could have gone to a patient a week earlier had we been advised. The only way is for the folk who are on the air to keep a watchful eye on those who are not, and thus enable us to make the necessary medical calls and reports. This service, of course, is always freely given by people of the Outback for their neighbours.[4]

Myra Blanch was willing to turn her hand to any task required of her. She remained at outback centres for however long she thought was in the interests of the local people. There are stories of her taking over the care of households during outbreaks of illness, administering to the sick, cleaning house, doing the cooking, acting as tutor to the children. 'She immediately took charge,' one woman wrote, 'and, after attending the patients, took to cleaning up the dust [a dust storm having raged the day prior], and, without flinching, turned to the cooking in no uncertain manner.'[5] On one occasion, when about to set out from an overnight stay at a homestead, she received a radio message. The folk from a nearby station could not get home that night – could she make a detour on her way back to the base and feed their fowls? It was only 50 kilometres out of her way so Sister Blanch was glad to oblige.

Sister Blanch took a particular interest in the welfare of the young, delighting in the presence of healthy happy outback children and lamenting the circumstances of those less favoured. 'The O'Reilly's have a family of six children, three of whom are away at school. Maureen is a quiet, shy little lass, who milks the cows and helps Mother about the house very efficiently, and rears motherless lambs as a hobby. The other children at home are aged four years and eighteen months – happy, healthy and wild. Garry, eighteen months, is never so happy as when, armed with a butcher's knife – the sight of which made my blood run cold – he goes out with his Father to kill a sheep.'[6]

Myra Blanch's itinerary depended on climatic conditions and transport opportunities but she endured hold-ups caused by bad weather with stoicism and moved from homestead to homestead in whatever form of conveyance was going her way. While she was at one homestead, a call came to visit another one nearby and, as there was no car or horse available, undaunted, she set out on foot. Eventually, in 1947, the section provided her with her own utility truck equipped with a portable transceiver. She adapted circumstances and conditions to suit herself and evolved her own uniform of shirt and slacks or breeches. When people in her jurisdiction hesitated to ask for help, Sister Blanch gave it notwithstanding. Conscious of the fact that most of the patients not removed to hospital were nursed by the women of the household, she regularly published 'Home Nursing Hints' in the section's magazine, giving advice on such matters as how to administer drugs from the medicine chest. Her instructions were quite stern – 'Your patient will probably not be at all keen on taking his fluids – he just "can't be bothered", and certainly will not be asking for them, so you must suggest it.'[7] She also conducted a weekly radio clinic which was very well received, particularly by the women.

Her surveys and reports on areas beyond the reach of the aircraft in the sparsely populated areas were invaluable and were considered ample justification of her appointment. By anyone's reckoning she would seem to have fulfilled the expectations outlined in her initial job description. She took leave from Broken Hill from 1951 to 1953 to study preventative medicine in England and, when she returned, stayed two more years. In 1953–54 she made a systematic survey of 260 station properties and outposts covering 400 000 square kilometres and an estimated population, excluding towns, of 2480 people. Her work, covering areas of interest such as public health and disease prevention, ante- and postnatal advice, and children's diets and immunisation, was incorporated into a valuable health survey of the network area which was subsequently published by the New South Wales Section.[8]

As the first nursing sister employed by the RFDS, Myra Blanch was well ahead of the regular recruitment of flight nurses which began in the 1960s. She was well ahead of her time, too, in her commitment to preventative health care, health education and health surveying, since the RFDS did not formally commit itself to a national primary health care role for another forty-eight years. This happened in 1993, with the adoption of a national health strategy entitled 'The Best for the Bush', which outlined a plan for the RFDS to extend its primary health care role into preventative health including women's health,

early childhood services, adolescent health, mental health, occupa-
tional health and Aboriginal and Torres Strait Islander health.

The RFDS has long recognised that the health of Aboriginal and
Torres Strait Islander people is of a standard considerably lower than
that of non-Indigenous Australians. As this group makes up approximately 40 per cent of RFDS patients, the Service has a significant role
to play in addressing the situation. One of its initiatives has been to
appoint Indigenous Health Liaison Officers who coordinate and
provide a range of health-related services that assist in the improvement of the health status of Aboriginal people.[9]

It is in areas of primary health care that nurses in the RFDS play
an important role. They conduct women's and children's health clinics
in isolated communities, together with the flying doctor who conducts
medically based health clinics. Some nurses have dedicated roles in
these areas; others serve concurrently as flight nurses. In 1945 the
Service employed one nurse. The current total is 114 nurses – 93 full
time and 21 part time.

The women's health nurses help ensure that women living in rural
and remote areas can access basic screening programs and health
information that many urban women take for granted. Women's
Health Nurse Jane Bryant includes among her tasks pap smears,
breast checks, antenatal care and contraceptive advice. She also strives
to become involved with the various communities. While recognising
that her work at each may be the same, to them the service is different
– each community is unique. 'It takes a while to build up a rapport
with clients and develop trust, particularly in communities like
Wilcannia or Menindee. The Aboriginal women there aren't very
proactive with their health care but there are valid reasons for that –
they are often dealing with issues that are simply not on the agenda
for people in other settings – so coming in for a pap smear may be
very low on their priority list.'

An important part of the nurses' work is to provide an environment in which clients feel comfortable chatting about sensitive issues
that they may not wish to discuss with friends or neighbours due to

confidentiality concerns. These are not necessarily medical matters but might be worries about a child or worries about life in general. 'So we do quite a bit of informal social work,' explains Jane. 'We talk to patients about their concerns and try to offer them useful strategies or practical assistance.'

The role of the RFDS children's health nurse focuses on children's primary health care and involves a range of procedures – advising on infant feeding, monitoring children's growth and development, implementing immunisation programs, conducting vision and hearing assessments and referring patients to specialist services as required. This work is carried out at defined rural health centres and also at bush clinics where there are no staff on site.

Child and Family Health Nurse Leesa Catford explains the requirements of the position:

> To do this job you have to be adaptable, to have a certain amount
> of resilience and to have a fair amount of trust in your colleagues
> and in yourself. Communication skills are quite important. I'm
> involved in helping others and empowering them – giving them
> the skills to see their strengths and to make the best of situations
> that are sometimes very difficult. The people I'm helping are
> parents and other health workers – everyone really. No one is an
> expert – everyone's got skills they can bring to a situation so it's a
> matter of giving people options and showing them there are ways
> forward even when things seem really gloomy around them.

The primary task is to assist communities to do things better as far as child and family health goes and this may involve tapping into existing facilities and linking up with other agencies outside the sphere of the RFDS. These nurses find the work immensely reward-ing, as Leesa comments: 'In big hospitals with a high patient turnover, it's hard to develop close ties. With flying doctor work, you become a part of the community and you can see how your work is improving people's lives.'

Today's RFDS is very much concerned with preventative practices so health promotion and education have increasingly become integrated into regular clinics. These programs have also been taken out of the medical setting and into the wider arena with health promotion stalls and illness-prevention activities introduced at field days and at events like rodeos and race meetings. In this way the RFDS can get their message across in an informal setting – perhaps by doing blood pressure checks or distributing pamphlets on issues such as heart health or diabetes – and reach people who might not otherwise attend a clinic.

17

No Place for a Woman

. . . .

When John Flynn began to establish his network of cottage hospitals, he intended that each should function from a central base and extend a mantle of care to the areas within their radius. In this regard he was unwittingly anticipating the process by which the Flying Doctor Service and eventually the nurses who became part of it would operate. Flynn's report to the Federal Assembly of the Presbyterian Church in 1912, *Northern Territory and Central Australia: A Call to the Church*, outlined his hopes for these isolated areas. One of these hopes was for the outback to become a more secure place for women to live. 'The first thing to do in any effort to uplift the tone of bush life is to give women a sense of security; in other words, to make child-bearing comparatively safe at the outposts.'[1] John Flynn believed strongly that the outback would not become adequately populated nor would the 'tone' be raised until this sense of security was achieved and women had the confidence to accompany their husbands into the remote areas where they lived and worked. With equal conviction he believed that an important way to make it safe for women was for female nurses to take up residence and provide nursing care and support.

Flynn had enormous confidence in the capabilities of women. His claim was that if something worthy needed to be done, it was simply a matter of telling the ladies what was wanted and then getting out of their way while they attended to it. For this reason he was keen to entice them into the Inland and in pursuit of that ideal made such an action sound like their patriotic duty. He wrote at the end of the First World War: 'By the time a girl is trained [in nursing], her parents are at least reconciled to her departure: most are keenly interested in it, and are proud to send forth their daughter for their country's sake. We care for the same country, and the same men, for whom all our nurses were recently ready to leave home. The soldiers are now filtering back to the far Inland, many of them, and they will need nurses as never before they enlisted.'[2]

Ever attendant to the practical side, Flynn went on to note that the salary paid to the nurse would be £100 per annum, with her companion receiving £52 per annum, plus fares, board and lodging. 'We hope, shortly,' he added reasonably, 'to finalise an arrangement by which we will pay heirs £300 in the event of her meeting a Willy Willy off Pilbara, or any other accident that should prove fatal, and interrupt remittances to those dependent on her.'[3]

Flynn was quite unrelenting when he wanted to recruit someone and to Nance Inglis, a young woman of his acquaintance whom he had earmarked as a possibility for AIM work, he wrote: 'By the way, if I may ask, what are your plans for life? I ask because we need some of God's best women in the bush as nurses and deaconesses. It is a long, dreary, difficult path to take in some respects, but it is interesting, noble, and satisfying. Perhaps I have said enough. Australia wants gentle, devoted women to take up Christ's work, and if you are free, and would like to help, I should be glad to hear'.[4] His plea was successful and Nance Inglis took up duty at the Port Hedland nursing home in 1919 and for many years after continued to give the AIM her staunch support.

In order to reach the hospitals to which they had been assigned, nurses made long journeys of days and sometimes weeks, initially by train or boat and then by horse, buggy or motor vehicle. When no other accommodation was available en route, they camped by the

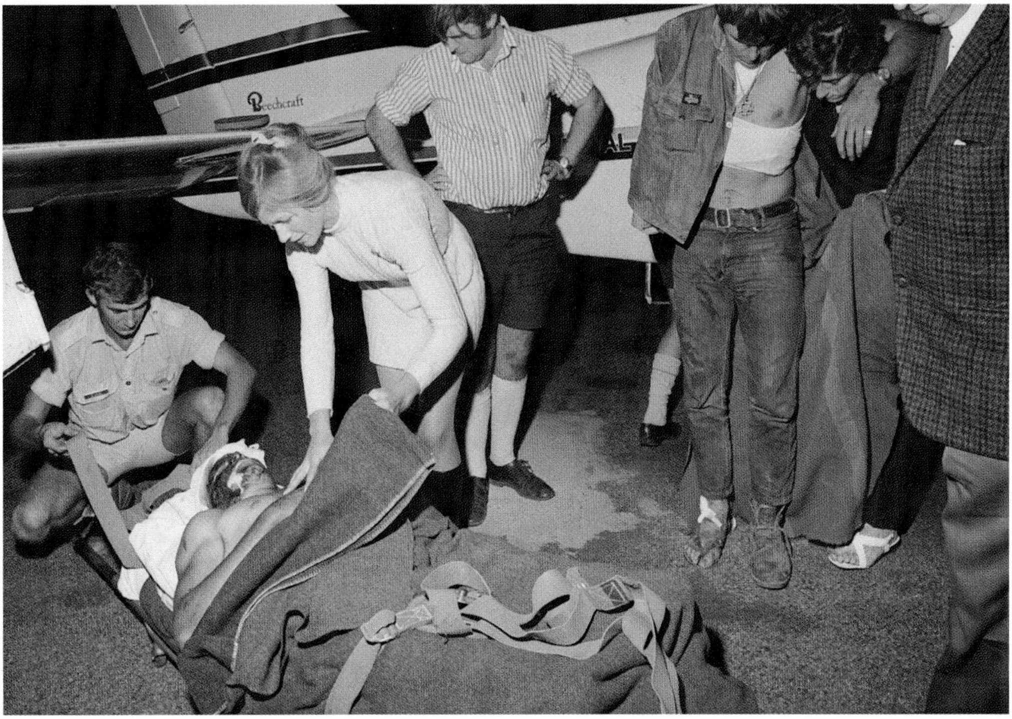

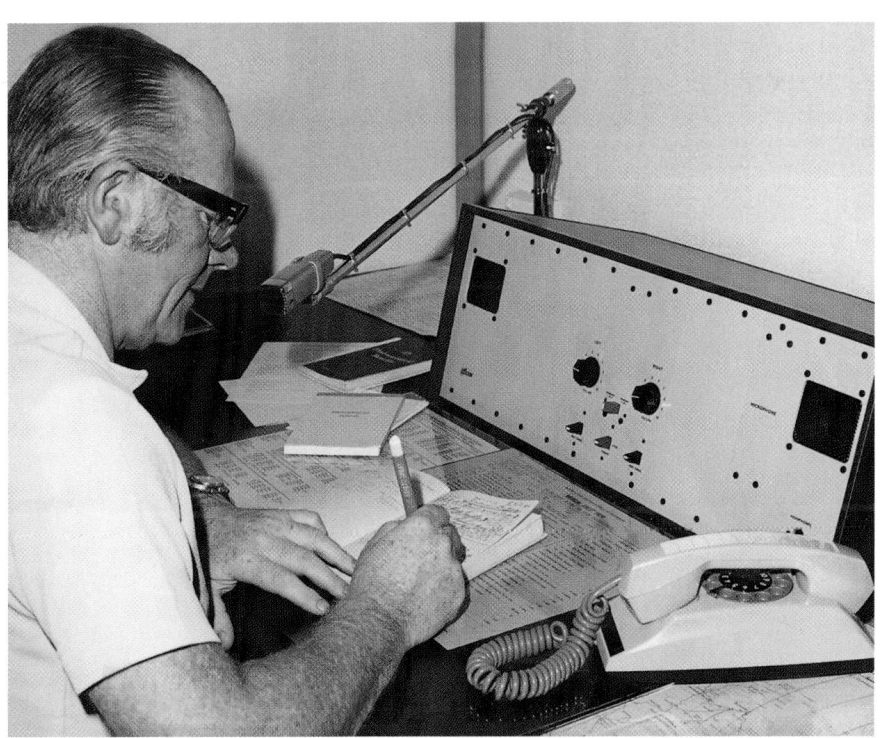

Robin Miller, nurse and pilot, attends a patient at Port Hedland

Dr Timothy O'Leary conducting a radio clinic — O'Leary served the RFDS in Queensland in numerous capacities over many years

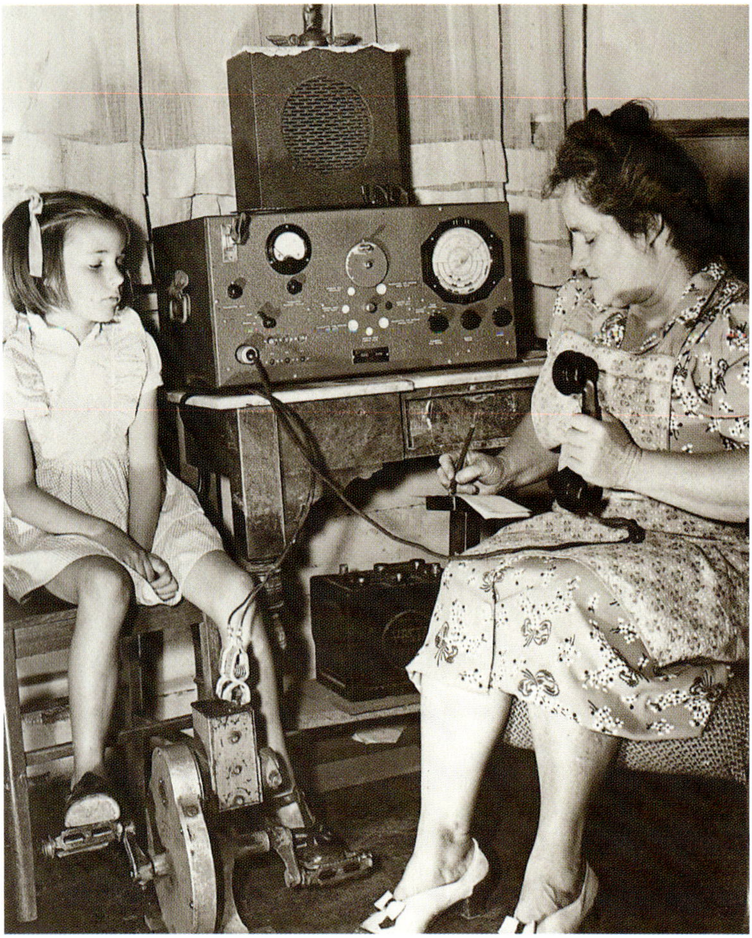

An outback girl pedals while her mother talks to the base using voice transmission, a huge improvement on morse code

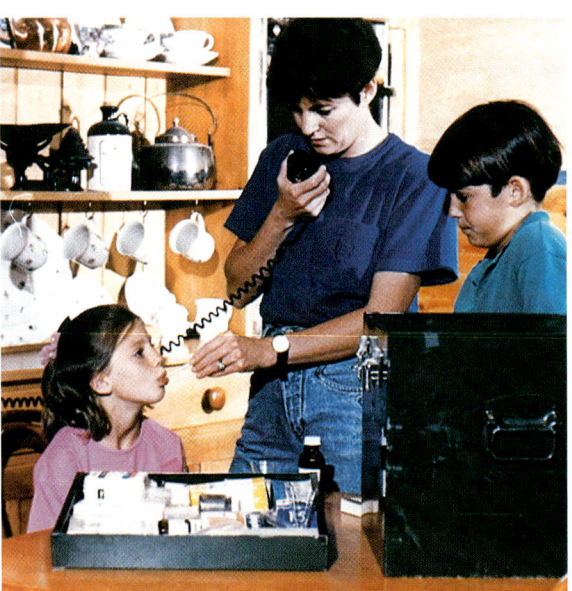

A mother administers to a child from a medical chest following instructions from the base doctor

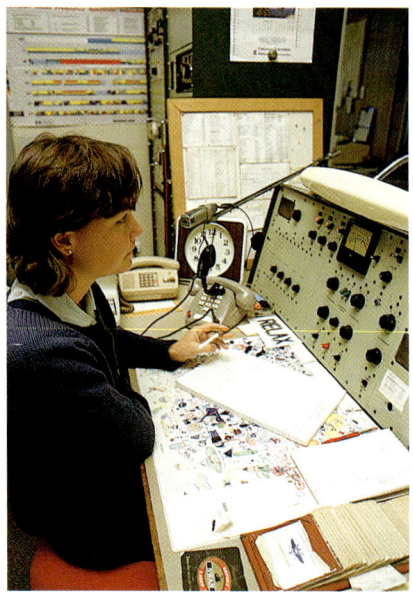

Alice Springs radio operator at work

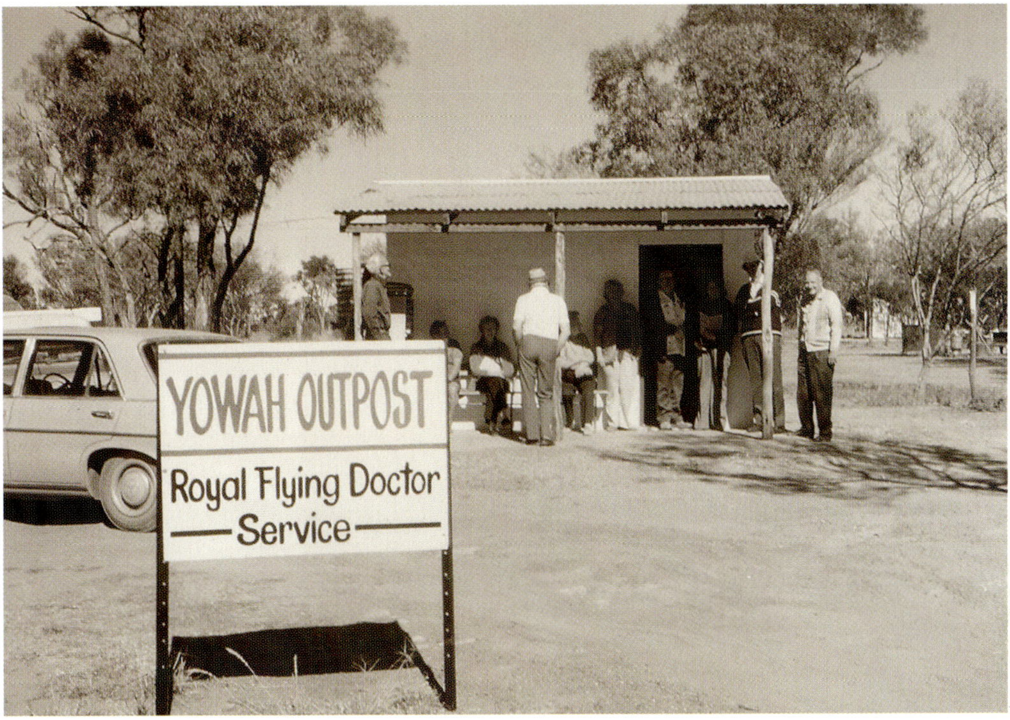

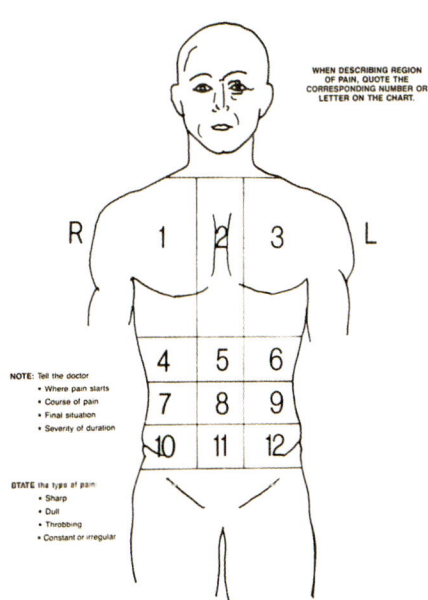

Patients line up to see the flying doctor at a bush clinic

WHEN DESCRIBING REGION
OF PAIN, QUOTE THE
CORRESPONDING NUMBER OR
LETTER ON THE CHART.

R   1   2   3   L

NOTE: Tell the doctor
• Where pain starts
• Course of pain
• Final situation
• Severity of duration

4   5   6

7   8   9

10   11   12

STATE the type of pain
• Sharp
• Dull
• Throbbing
• Constant or irregular

'Where does it hurt?' Body charts
help doctors to pinpoint ailments
from a distance.

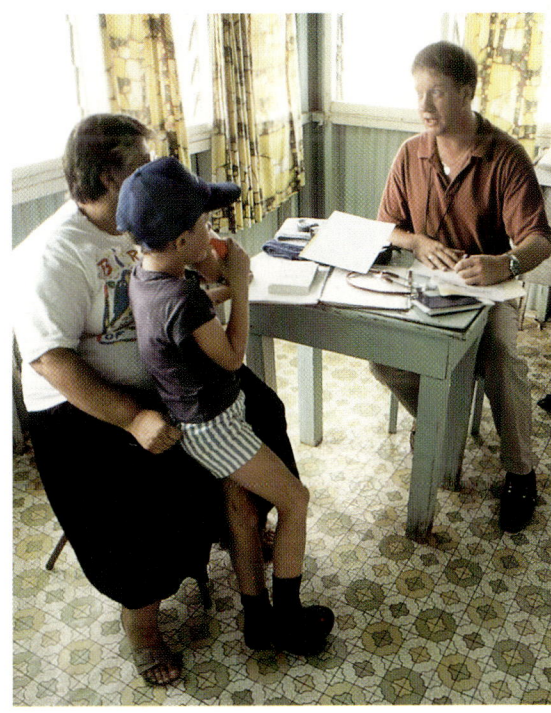

A Queensland doctor consults with a mother and
child

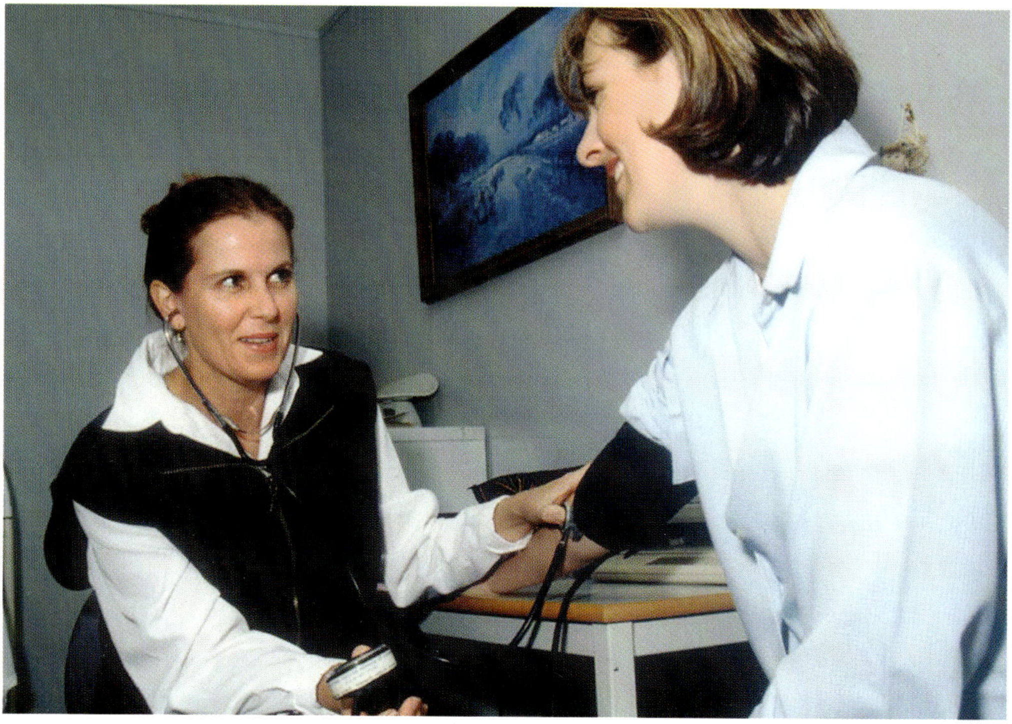

Women's Health nurse, Jane Bryant, consults with a patient

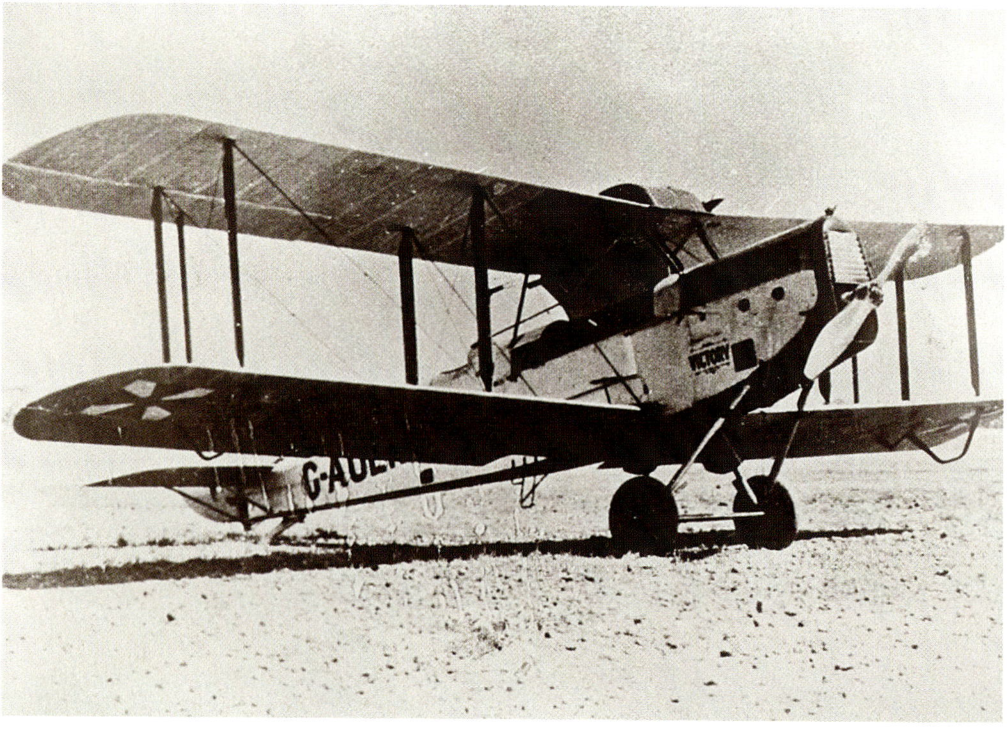

Victory, chartered from Qantas, was the plane used by the Aerial Medical Service for its inaugural flight on 17 May 1928 from Cloncurry

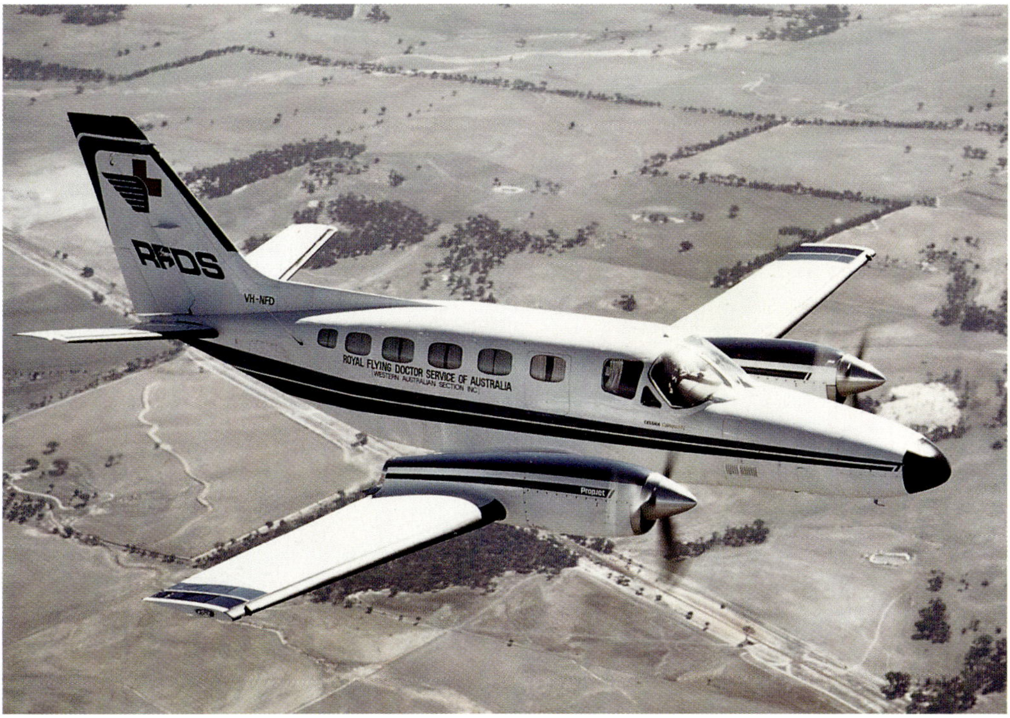

Aerial shot of Cessna Conquest in Western Australia; the Cessna Conquest was the Section's first turbine aircraft and marked the beginning of a new era in medical aviation for the Section.

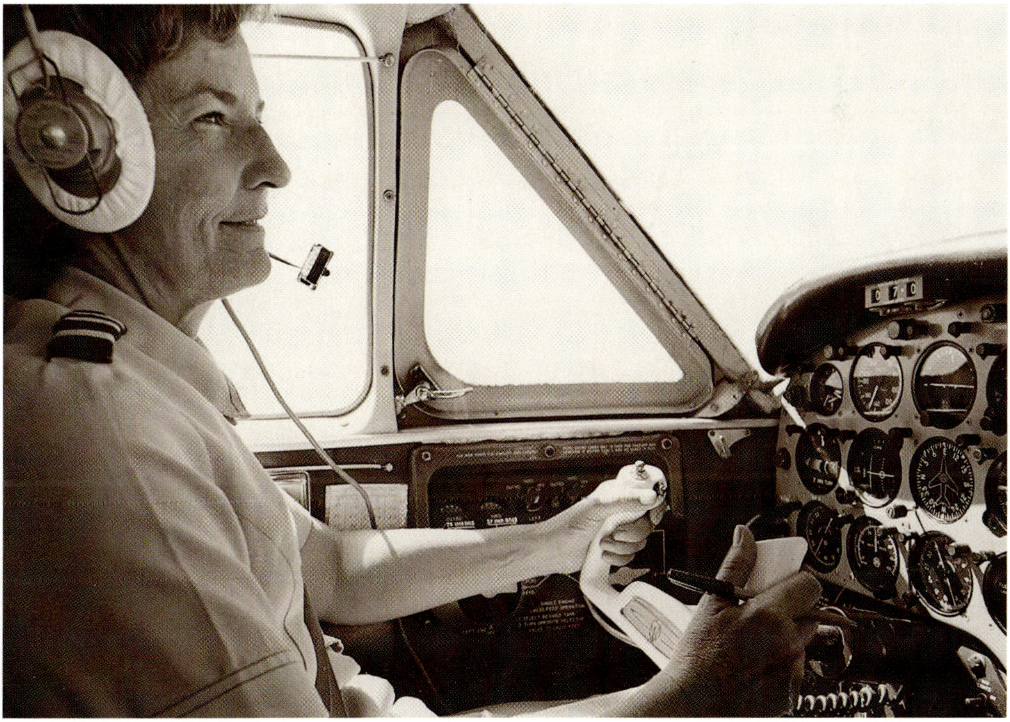

Captain Beth Garrett, first woman RFDS pilot, at the controls in Queensland

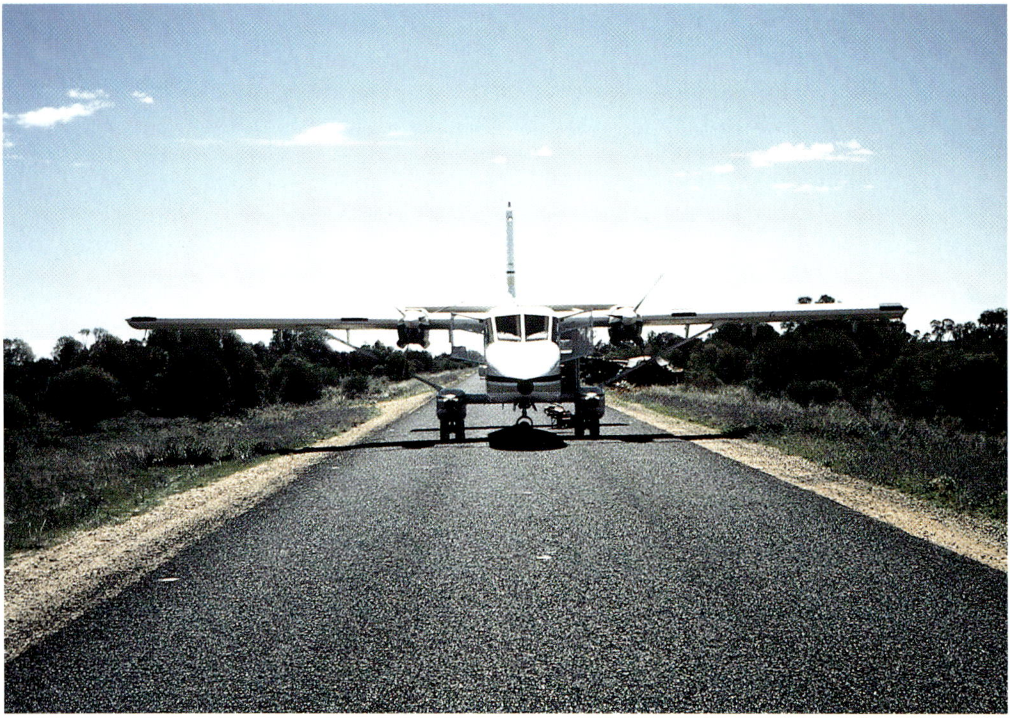

With no suitable airstrip available, an RFDS plane lands on a road

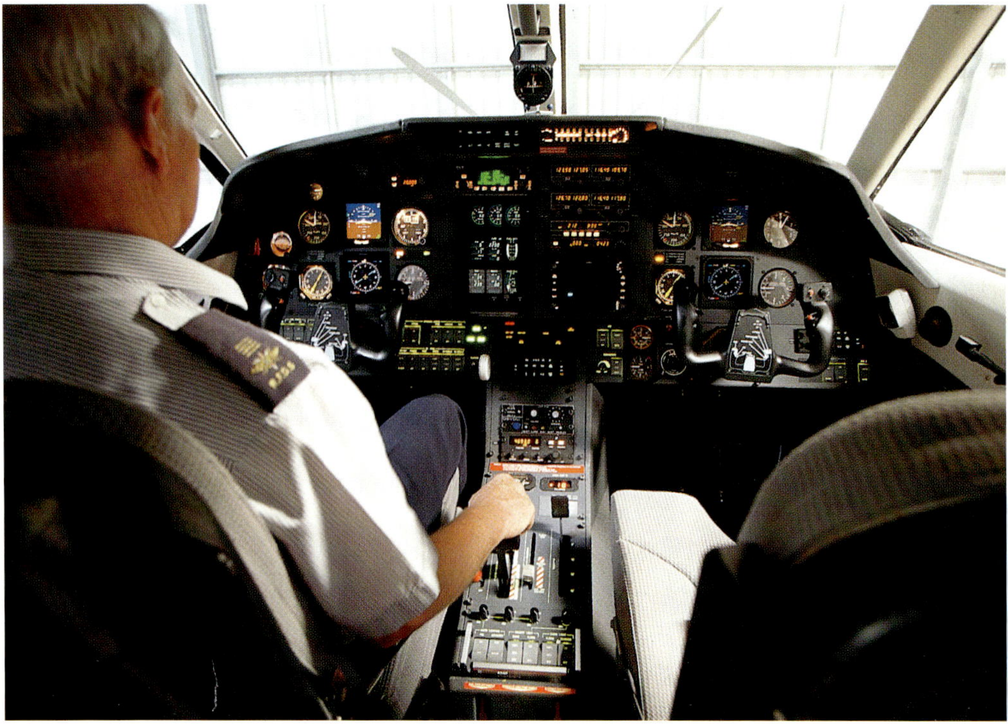

Cockpit of a Pilatus PC12, the newest type of plane to be included in the RFDS fleet

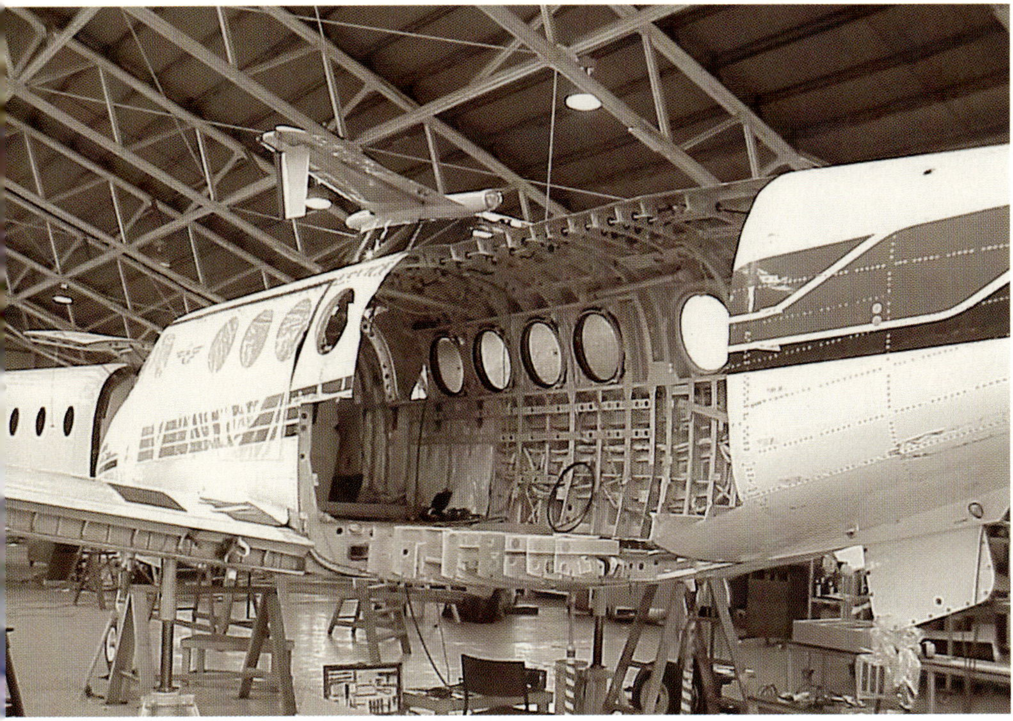

It takes months of work to transform an aircraft into a flying intensive care unit

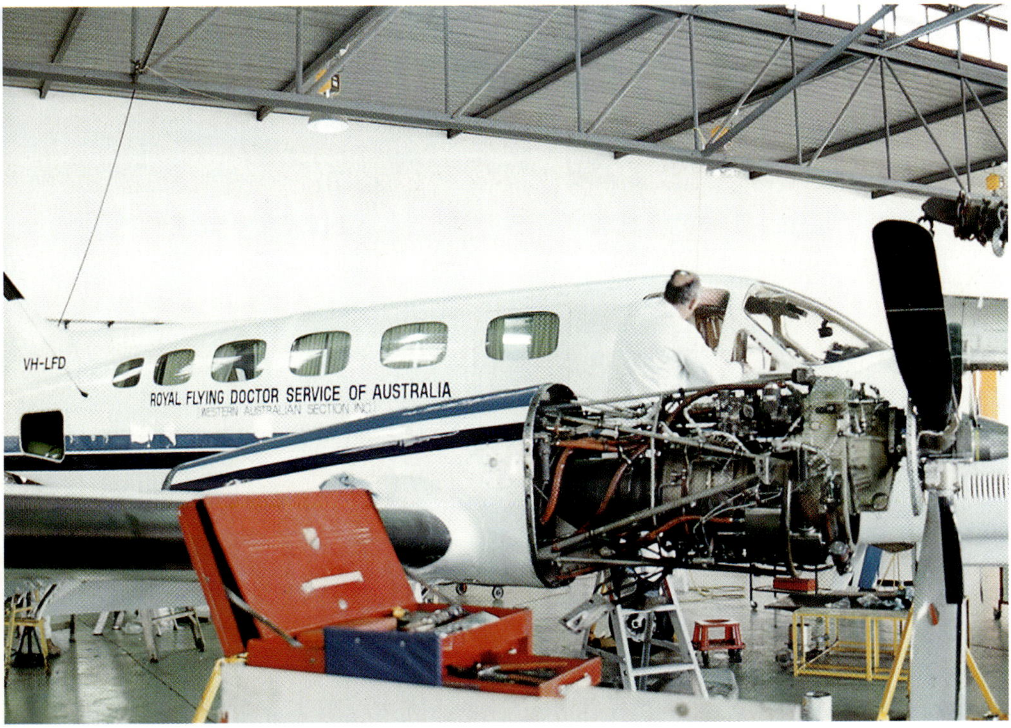

A Cessna Conquest undergoing maintenance at port

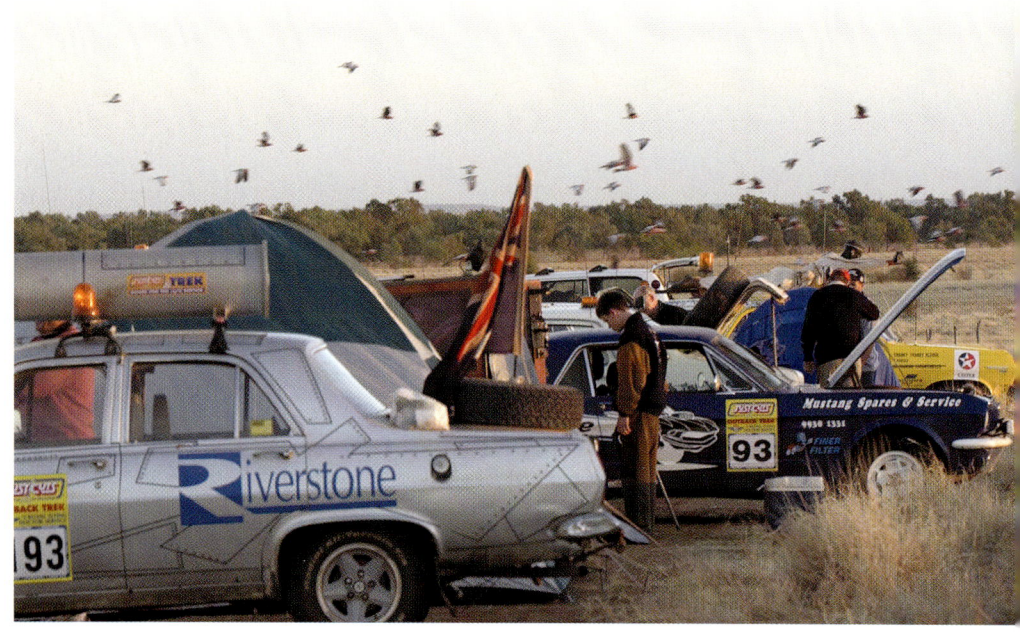

The Outback Car Trek is a major fundraiser for the RFDS

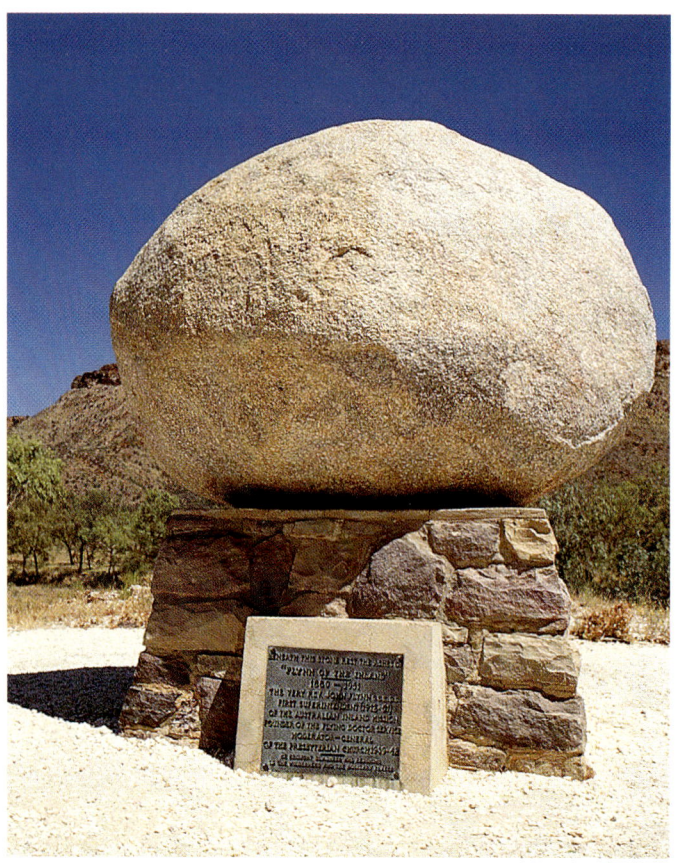

The rock depicted here atop John Flynn's grave at Alice Springs was returned to its custodians, the Kaytetye people, in September 1999 and replaced with a similar rock offered by the Arrernte people

track. This account concerns a replacement nurse destined for the
Dunbar hostel. At the time of the report she was staying at a homestead following heavy rain, waiting for an opportunity to get to her
new posting across the river.

> As the time drew near for Sister Jeffcoate to leave, Sister Jones
> decided she must make an attempt at all costs to reach the
> nursing home. Leaving the homestead by truck, Sister and her
> companion managed to get the truck to the other side of the
> river, then rowed across the main channel, which is at present
> very high, with a strong current. Leaving the boat they had to
> walk through cane grass to their shoulders and mud ankle-deep.
> From the cane grass to the next bank they had to swim for some
> distance, then Sister walked the remaining five miles alone to
> Dunbar, through long grass, mud and water.[5]

Such a trip would surely have caused most people to return home
immediately. But the AIM nurses were made of sterner stuff. There
are many anecdotes similar to this one and it is a tribute to their
tenacity that these women not only endured the hardship of reaching
their destination, but stayed on to grapple with additional problems
after their arrival. And having served their one- or two-year term,
undaunted, they sometimes signed up for another hostel in a different
area or married into the locality and signed up for a lifetime in the
bush.

Most of the nurses went to hostels that were already established.
However, nurses like Jean Finlayson, who went to Alice Springs in
1916, did so at Flynn's request, to report on the advisability of establishing a hostel there in the future. (The hostel at Alice Springs was
eventually completed in 1926.) Lacking a dedicated building in which
to live and work, Sister Finlayson carried out her nursing tasks in the
most rudimentary accommodation.

This was also the case for the unique group of itinerant nurses
termed 'border sisters' in the Innamincka area. The first was Sister

Marjorie Kinnear. She had no permanent residence but was accommodated in turn at the three main homesteads of the border region. She and her successors nursed their scattered population over a scope of some 18 130 square kilometres. They worked without the benefit of a hospital and its amenities, with the nearest doctor 805 kilometres away and no telegraph or railway within 644 kilometres. Drugs had to be ordered four or five months in advance, and during epidemics of illness, supplies were soon exhausted. Contacting the nurse was a dilemma when an emergency arose at one station and the nurse was tending a patient at another. Then the decision had to be made as to which of the two cases was the most pressing. Ultimately the complicated nature of this type of nursing was acknowledged and a more secure arrangement was made in the establishment of the nursing home at Innamincka.

Even with a hostel to work in the nurses battled with a variety of obstacles. They were extremely well-trained women, accustomed to the disciplined working environment of city hospitals which featured modern amenities and specialised medical backup. To nurse in professional isolation with constant shortages of food, medicine and equipment was a trial in itself. With drought, floods, dust storms, thunderstorms, heat, cold, flies, mosquitos, snakes, spiders and rat plagues added to the mix, their difficulties intensified. Any one of these would severely try the patience of the average person – to endure several of them at once must surely elevate these women to hero status.

As well as attending to patients both at the hostel and at considerable distances, the nurses washed, cleaned, cooked, made their own bread, milked goats or cows, raised hens, taught Sunday school to the children, distributed books and reading matter and despatched telegrams when the transceiver became available. When hostel wards were full, they nursed the overflow of patients in beds placed in the sitting room or on the verandah. If motor transport was not available, nurses who had never before sat a saddle rode to their patients on horseback. After one such 48-kilometre trip, old hands cheerfully informed

Sister Burchill, an inexperienced rider, that she would be eating her tea 'off the mantlepiece' and this proved to be the case! Sister Giles of Beltana spoke of dealing with patients affected by the Depression of the 1930s. 'We have lots of patients in hospital who have been out of work for months. They are generally in a bad way when they reach us – having had no decent food; consequently they take twice the amount of care and attention, and are in hospital longer than they would otherwise need to be.'[6] And during the war the AIM sisters at Fitzroy Crossing and Halls Creek were called upon to give medical advice by radio in place of doctors who had joined the services.[7]

Some of the nursing sisters helped to bury the dead and, in the absence of any more appropriate person to officiate, conducted the burial service, using the words from Flynn's *Bushman's Companion*. As this account from Halls Creek illustrates, in caring for their patients, the sisters stayed true to the doctrine that the hostel and its facilities were to be available to all, irrespective of colour, creed or nationality:

> Our poor old patient, Esau, died on 7 January, poor old fellow. He had been an inmate for three years, so the hospital was his home. He was very old and felt the heat greatly. Esau was a Mahommedan. The Afghans held a service and attended to the funeral arrangements. There were quite a number of men camped about 7 miles out, so they all came in. One was a priest in their religion, so he held a service in the ward, and then the burial took place at 9 pm.[8]

A constant problem for the nursing sisters was to provide suitable food for convalescing patients, especially in areas where supplies were delivered infrequently and before the advent of refrigerators. One border sister reported from one of the cattle stations within her jurisdiction:

> A young daughter of the hospitable host and hostess had been seriously ill with typhoid. With the help of a good medical

journal, she was recovering, but needed a special diet. There was
no milk, no butter, no fruit or vegetables nearer than 400 miles,
as it was the dry season. The only milking goat had gone dry and
a neighbour nearly 100 miles away had another milking goat
who also went dry. The only diet suitable was jellies made after
the sun went down and hung in a tin billy down the well and
eaten before sunrise; a few young chickens were killed and with
the added broth, the patient recovered.[9]

To augment the standard diet of meat and more meat, nurses
planted vegetable gardens and fruit trees which, if they survived the
rigours of local climatic conditions, were much appreciated by those
who came after. One nurse wrote from Beltana, 'There has not been
any rain here for some time, and the ground is hard and dry. Our
garden was looking its best about a month ago. The cauliflowers are
finished, and the blight is attacking the other vegetables'.[10] Another,
from Alice Springs, lamented, 'Fine vegetable gardens are drooping
because of the storm. Cabbages, tomatoes, onions, silver beet and
grape vines all flat and wilted'.[11]

Insufficient rainfall was a constant trial. Water at Halls Creek when
scarce had to be carted from a well at a distance from the hostel and
at Oodnadatta it arrived too hot from the artesian bores to provide
refreshment. From Port Hedland came this unfortunate story: 'We are
still longing for rain, and are much grieved, because it looks as though
our gardens and trees will have to die; in fact, Sister bought 100
gallons of water herself today in order to keep some young poinciana
trees going until they spread their roots down to the moisture.'[12]
When water supplies permitted, nurses nurtured their lawns, trees and
shrubs in an attempt to make the hostel surroundings more attractive
for patients and visitors.

In addition to their medical duties, an important part of the AIM
nurse's brief was to contribute to the well-being of the locals by offering the hostel as a haven where both locals and travellers could rest

and visit. The nurses became the nucleus of their communities' social life. Sometimes they simply provided a chat and a cup of tea. At other times they hosted small gatherings, morning teas, bridge parties, dances, musical evenings, and importantly, Christmas celebrations for the children. The Christmas party became a feature of the hostels, with the nurses working tirelessly to put up decorations and provide party food. They encouraged supporters in the cities to donate gifts for the children which, if they arrived in time, were distributed by a local dressed as Santa Claus, sweltering in the December temperatures.

Whether it was the humid heat of the tropical north or the very dry heat of Central Australia, the summer months had a debilitating effect on the nurses who came to their postings from the cooler climates of coastal towns and cities. Elizabeth Burchill, in her book *Innamincka*, makes an interesting comment about the weather and about the locals' attitude to the nurses' imaginative way of dealing with it:

> The Inland weather usually demanded that we wear a minimum
> of clothing, although the crisp early mornings and evenings of
> the winter months made cardigans a necessity. We wore cotton
> uniforms all day and stockings, too, because Inlanders were
> surprisingly conventional about such things. They frowned on
> our early habit of donning bathing suits to do the laundry, even
> when the heat was at its worst.[13]

The Inlanders were a stalwart group who made the most of their living conditions and improved on them imaginatively. Jessie Litchfield, an identity in the Northern Territory from her arrival at the beginning of the twentieth century, was prominent in helping to formulate Flynn's ideas about the needs of isolated communities. She observed:

> Out bush you simply had to be able to turn your hand to
> anything. I have soled my own shoes, mended leaks in

frying-pans and saucepans with the soldering iron and flux, have
helped my husband build the bark humpies we lived in, (or
pulled them down and rebuilt them if they did not suit my taste).
I have made my own bread, and lemon butter and potted meat.
Made chilli drinks from the chillies grown round the house,
made ginger beer, went out prospecting with my husband if he
wanted to test a likely spot, taught my children for part of the
time by correspondence methods – in short, turned my hand to
anything and everything, from building a table to planning a
fancy-dress for a child to wear.[14]

Brave and resourceful themselves, the nurses found the Inlanders
even more so, and this went beyond admiration of their ability to
manage day-to-day exigencies with limited resources. The sisters also
admired the ingenuity of the people they attended in medical situations. A nursing sister at Halls Creek was called to attend a man who
had broken an arm and two ribs. When she arrived at his camp she
found the patient on a bed made up of branches and the remains of
an anthill. His brother had fashioned splints from bark, and had bound
his ribs with a towel.[15] As the nurses used *The Bushman's Companion*
to guide them through a burial service, perhaps the bushmen who
could splint broken limbs received their tuition from the same source.
The nurses were inspired also by the fortitude of those who endured
long arduous trips with horrific injuries to reach the hostels, and by
the Aboriginal people they nursed who endured treatment without
complaint which, as the nurses often commented, was 'typical of
their race'.

Inlanders were often equipped with a medical journal which they
desperately consulted when someone was sick and which they inter-
preted with a degree of guesswork. Arch Grant, in *Camel Train &
Aeroplane*, tells the story of a sick miner in the wolfram fields at
Hatches Creek in the Northern Territory: 'When a member of the
camp, Dick Brown, became ill, with the aid of a doctor's book, Skipper

[AIM patrol padre] and some of the others tried to diagnose his complaint, but could only reduce the variables to "apoplexy, appendicitis, internal rupture or strain but which of these it was, we could not decide". Brown took the matter into his own hands and shot himself.'[16]

The nursing sisters in their cottage hospitals took away some of the burden of care from those who no doubt rejoiced to be free of it. Nonetheless, death still stalked the Inlanders. The perennial problem of distance continued to thwart the nurses' efforts to reach patients in time to avert tragedies. Prior to widespread immunisation programs being instigated, epidemic diseases like tuberculosis, diphtheria, scarlet fever and typhoid took their toll. Common complaints such as colds and measles assumed alarming proportions and seriousness in isolated communities, particularly among Aboriginal communities. There are frequent stories of Aboriginal people with high fever during measles epidemics taking on their own treatment. This account from Fitzroy Crossing illustrates.

> The Sisters have been very busy indeed, on account of the measles epidemic in the West Kimberleys. This illness takes a very severe form with the natives, who require close supervision in hospital. One Aboriginal mother and babe, although running high temperatures, were found on several occasions cooling off in the river or wandering along its banks, and were restored to the ward without further ado, the incident being regarded with much merriment by them. Both Trixie and her baby made a good recovery.[17]

Another common injury among Aboriginal patients was burns – the result of huddling too close to fires in the cold weather. At Fitzroy Crossing a sister wrote: 'A young Aboriginal girl was brought in from one of the stations suffering from severe burns, as she had fallen into the fire. She was in a shocking condition, but after treatment quickly improved. She is very brave and never complains although her suffering must be great.'[18]

Apart from the more serious epidemic diseases, the nurses dealt with quite a range of conditions which, in the absence of modern drugs, required careful nursing to overcome. They mentioned skin infections, stomach upsets, sore throats, boils, broken bones, sprains, snakebite and the ubiquitous problems of 'sore eyes' which seemed to afflict everyone and which the nurses blamed on the presence of flies.

Toothache was a common complaint also, with the result that a large part of the nurse's job involved dentistry, mainly extracting teeth that might have been saved had there been a trained dentist available. Judging from the numerous reports from the nurses about this particular service there must have scarcely been a single Inlander who still had a full set of teeth. The nurses all received some elementary instruction in dental care as part of their preparation for bush nursing, and this was enough for people in the bush to travel hundreds of miles to have a raging toothache relieved.

The sisters even took impressions for dentures with material sent from dentists in the capital cities, then returned the impressions and waited with bated breath to see if they had managed a fit. In the absence of proper material for the task, resourcefulness was called for. Elizabeth Burchill had to remove a young woman's upper eye teeth which were supporting a dental plate and needed to take an impression of her gums.

> The small daughter of the house brought me a cardboard box
> containing a quantity of coloured wax made up into sticks. I took
> two of them and softened them in steam. Soon they were pliable
> enough to push into my patient's mouth. The wax cooled,
> hardened and left a clear cut impression of the gums that
> exceeded my wildest dreams. Later the young woman's denture
> and the impression were sent to the dentist ... In a few weeks the
> completed work was returned and, back at Innamincka, word
> came to me from the patient that 'everything fits perfectly'.[19]

Eventually the inadequacy of dental treatment in the outback led to discussions by the Federal Council in 1944 of the possibility of a flying dentist being appointed so that a formal dental plan could be instigated. Mitigating factors included the difficulty of transporting cumbersome dental equipment by plane. The Queensland Section was the first to put the idea into practice with a Flying Dental Service inaugurated in 1946–47 in Charleville. The first dentist, GP Castles, went around to stations in the area and was picked up by RFDS aircraft on their routine flights. During the year he examined 411 patients and performed 372 extractions and 683 other dental operations.[20] It was proposed that flying dentists be appointed in other sections as soon as possible. This proposal was thwarted by the paucity of dentists willing to leave thriving city practices to carry out the work. Various schemes in other sections were implemented at different times, some involving dentists travelling in a fully equipped van rather than by plane. As the scheme developed, there were fewer extractions required as the efficacy of previous visits began to take effect.

The New South Wales Section began a dental service in 1960. This was arranged with the New South Wales Health Department who provided the dentist, while the RFDS provided the plane and the clinics in which the dentist could operate. Using specially designed lightweight equipment suitable for carrying on an aircraft, a dentist and nurse toured the Service's network during the school holidays. The following year the service was established on a permanent basis. It is on record that Dr Bob Burns, the section's first flying dentist, one day famously completed 120 fillings, with pilot Vic Cover working the treadle for the drill. Today dental clinics are a well-established part of the RFDS with education about oral health and preventative care rather than repairs being the primary focus.

18

Nurses in Full Flight

. . . .

The presence of the nursing sisters had the effect that Flynn had hoped for, and as the years passed, a steady stream of women came to settle in the outback and raise their families there. As more and more babies were successfully delivered by the nurses, there was increased confidence in applying to them for help. There are accounts of nurses being congratulated by doctors for delivering babies safely when a baby's untimely arrival meant there was insufficient time for the mother to travel to a major hospital.

Although the nurses recounted their stories of hardship with relish, they were also quick to point out the positives – the friendships made, the generosity of the locals who shared what they had and helped the nurses in innumerable ways, the visits to station homesteads, the excursions – picnicking, boating, swimming, fishing – and the grandeur of the wide-open spaces that became their living environment.

The nursing sisters carried out their tasks with courage and good humour. Their ability to see the funny side of situations made their stories entertaining and engaging. If they had doubts about why they had gone to these remote outposts or misgivings about their ability to really make a difference, they seemed not to show it. There is little to suggest in their reports to the AIM published in various magazines that they were ever other than totally dedicated to their work and resigned to tolerating whatever hardships came their way. A feature was their non-judgmental attitude. Medical conditions that were self-inflicted or resulted from neglect or ignorance were treated with the same loving kindness as any other complaint. Such was the standard of work of the initial trailblazers that nurses who followed after often did so because they were inspired by the example that had been set.

By the time the Flying Doctor Service was airborne, there were eleven nursing homes operating in Queensland, Western Australia, South Australia and the Northern Territory. In that year the sisters treated 581 in-patients, 1797 outpatients and 60 dental patients.[1] While the sisters did not act formally as flight nurses, being employed by the AIM, they were nonetheless very much part of the Flying Doctor Service, using the radio network to consult the flying doctor about patients or to organise the evacuation of patients by plane to nearby hospitals. During the 1940s there were indications from the nurses that they were beginning to fly themselves, accompanying patients to hospitals at the request of doctors. This account from Fitzroy Crossing in 1945: 'We had a patient about whom we were very worried recently, and Dr Roberts sent an ambulance plane to take him to Broome. We found there was no medical attendant, and, as it was my nursing week, I had to accompany him to Broome. There doctor found it necessary to send him on to Perth, and asked me to accompany him.'[2]

In the following year, a nurse from Dunbar hostel was thrilled to realise a long-held wish to visit the various mission stations in Cape York Peninsula. She went by plane, and assisted the doctor to immunise the children against whooping cough. In 1949, again at Fitzroy Crossing, a sister writes of receiving five Aboriginal people at the hostel who had been camped beneath a tree that was struck by lightning.

> It was dreadful business and the place was in a state of chaos for a
> while when they all arrived with dozens of relatives. They were
> all badly burnt and shocked and the smell of burnt charred flesh
> was dreadful. All their clothes and belongings were burnt and one

boy received a fractured base of the skull – and is very sick. No part of the tree fell so we think, perhaps, the lightning struck his head. I contacted doctor by wireless the following morning, and he sent a plane out with instructions for me to go with three of them. I took the fractured skull and the two worst burns.[3]

Formalising the concept of a flying sister was raised in 1946 when the section council suggested that the Kimberley region should have a flying sister based at Halls Creek to travel in the plane when the doctor was unavailable.[4] This suggestion was not acted on but nurses from various state health departments or government hospitals continued to be seconded to act as flight nurses, in addition to their normal duties at the hospitals where they worked. In 1950 the West Australian Health Department appointed Sister Lucy Garlick to the area served by the Wyndham base to attend to the welfare of the women and children throughout the Kimberley area. Her work was similar to that of Myra Blanch in Broken Hill. In 1952 the Victorian Section (responsible for the Kimberley area) agreed to be responsible for Sister Garlick's fare if arrangements could be made for her periodically to visit outposts on the doctor's round.[5] Garlick also features in RFDS history for her invention of the body chart which was subsequently used by flying doctors in their radio diagnoses.

Flight sisters were not used by the sections on a regular basis until the 1960s. Sister Marie Osborn was one of the first to be appointed and worked from the Derby base in the Kimberleys. When interviewed by Jill Newlands for an oral history project, 'The Nurses' Story', about how she got the job, Marie Osborn replied that it was because she was already there, had some tropical nursing experience and weighed eight stone, important since the aeroplane operated under stringent weight restrictions. Sister Osborn describes a typical day as follows: 'We took off at five o'clock every morning and I'd get up at half past three and then whiz over and make the lunches, collect the patient at half past four and we'd take off at five o'clock, and sometimes we flew until last light. Later on the restrictions were passed that they weren't allowed to fly as long as that, for which I was duly grateful.'[6]

Flight nurses during the history of the RFDS have recorded some traumatic experiences while carrying out their duties. One story involved an elderly man who had fallen after a drinking spree and injured his head. As a precaution, it was decided to evacuate him to hospital. During the flight the patient released his restraining straps, got off the stretcher and attempted to open the door of the aircraft. He meant no harm – he was simply trying to return to the pub! After a courageous struggle the flight nurse on board managed to sedate him and return him safely to his stretcher while the pilot, wearing earphones, remained blissfully unaware of the drama being played out in the back of the plane.[7]

The role of the flight nurses has evolved over time and expanded exponentially. An interesting development is that men are now involved in this work just as women are now involved as doctors and pilots, initially the province of men.

One of the reasons for the emergence of the role of a dedicated flight nurse was the desirability of training nurses in the particular requirements of working in an aviation transport environment.

Senior Flight Nurse Susan Markwell notes that the vital difference between a nurse in a hospital setting and one on board an aircraft is that flight nurses must be well briefed on all aspects of aircraft safety and have a knowledge of aviation physiology. 'You need to know your gas laws,' explains Susan. 'Gas expands when you go up so if you've got any space occupying lesions, that is, bubbles of air caught in your gut or your lungs, they're going to increase in size as you go up. So you have to be mindful of this and you would then ask the pilot to fly at sea-level pressure which gives you a much lower cabin altitude.'

Today, based on the judgment of the doctor authorising the flight, approximately 80 per cent of medical evacuations are made with only a flight nurse and pilot on board so their responsibilities are considerable. RFDS nurses are highly qualified. They must be regis- tered as a general nurse and midwife in the appropriate state; have significant relevant postgraduate experience including critical care; and be competent in procedural skills including advanced life support, emergency management of trauma, IV insertion, and interpretation of ECG and defibrillation.[8]

The flight nurse's role begins prior to flight with the pre-flight assessment and preparation for transport, extends throughout the phase of transport, and ends with the handover of the patient to the nominated facility.[9]

Nurse Manager David White makes this point: 'Because most of our flights are nurse only it is my role to make sure that the nurses are adequately skilled for that role. They have to be very experienced in emergency nursing, very experienced in critical care and well proficient in midwifery skills. Because we're taking the hospital to the patient and we can't fit five or six staff members on board, the one person we do take has to have all these skills.'

There are other personal characteristics required of a flight nurse which cannot be written into a job description – tenacity, emotional and mental flexibility, the ability to work long, irregular hours, to work in a team across disciplines and in a constrained environment, and, as flight nurses will point out – a sense of humour.

It is a tough job so why do they do it? David White provides the answer:

> We've flown into places late at night and people in the bush have
> told me, 'There's no sweeter sound in the world than the sound
> of engines coming' because their little one has asthma or their
> husband has severe chest pain. And they're terrified. There's no
> help within 1000 kilometres and we're it. Because when someone
> dies out here, it affects the whole community. They're tough
> people out here – they're not interested in malarky. They say
> with a tear in their eye, 'You saved my son'. You get that in large
> hospitals too but it's something extra here because if we don't
> turn up, they have nothing. That's a great feeling.

THE DOCTOR
TAKES WINGS

19

Early remedies

. . . .

An advertisement appeared in the *Medical Journal of Australia* of 24 December 1927 in the 'Medical Appointments Vacant' section which was an Australian first. A flying doctor was sought to join the AMS in Cloncurry, to commence in May of the following year. The terms of appointment for the doctor provided a salary of £1000 per annum without board, life insurance cover of £2000, and travelling expenses and board when away from the base. (An interesting comparison can be made with an advertisement seventy-five years later for a flying doctor in Western Australia offering six weeks annual leave, two weeks study leave, house and utilities, vehicle, relocation costs, superannuation and salary packaging.)[1] Twenty-two people applied for the position and Dr Kenyon St Vincent Welch was the candidate chosen.

Although existing air services in the area had already been used informally for taking the sick or injured to hospitals, there was no doctor dedicated to such missions and the missions were at a cost that few could afford. Hudson Fysh, in *Qantas Rising*, recounts the story of such a mercy mission in 1924 which he claimed could have been a first.

Dr Michod [of Longreach] contacted me. Would I fly out urgently to Corona station, 58 miles away, to bring in Mrs Armstrong, wife of the manager, who was imminently expecting a baby? I must admit that I hesitated, being most apprehensive that Mrs Armstrong would have the baby during our hour's journey from the station to the hospital. Under pressure from the doctor I agreed to do the job, providing all the stations over which we would pass were notified, so that I could land quickly in case of emergency.

The extraordinary circumstances of this trip were that some years before, when no aeroplanes were available, Mr Armstrong's first wife was due to have a baby. Down came the floods, cutting them off from medical help, and mother and child died. Mr Armstrong had married again and now the same dread position had arisen.

I landed the old BE2E on the beaten-down roadway near Corona station and, keeping my engine running, soon had Mrs Armstrong sitting up in the little passenger seat in front. Off we took, and in one hour according to my logbook had completed the journey to Longreach, where Dr Michod was waiting on the aerodrome to receive us. All was well and a baby girl was duly born in the Longreach hospital – perhaps Australia's first baby whose mother had been flown into hospital just prior to giving birth.[2]

When the plans for the AMS were being formulated, a simple air ambulance scheme such as this had been proposed but never acted on, as it was thought inadvisable for a pilot to have to supervise a patient in addition to flying the plane. Judging from the disquiet his medical mission had caused him, Fysh would no doubt have thoroughly endorsed this way of thinking! It was decided instead that there should always be a medical attendant on the flight. This was a result of recommendations from the AIM's chief medical adviser, Dr George

Simpson, who had prepared a report in the lead-up to the Cloncurry operation based on his observations of what would be needed. He pointed out that a medical practitioner in attendance would enable an evaluation to be made as to whether the patient could safely make a flight and for treatment to be given while in the air – including presumably, delivering a baby. Simpson advised, 'In case of air sickness and vomiting it may be necessary to clear the mouth. The injection of morphine may be needed for patients after accident. Stimulants may be needed. Adjustments of splints and dressings may be necessary. The pilot would have his own responsibilities and could not be expected to worry about the welfare of the passenger.'[3] This practice continues today with every medical flight carrying either a doctor or a flight nurse to supervise the needs of the patient.

A further stipulation was that the flying doctor would have no right of private practice but would be encouraged to help out at various hospitals when not on flying duty, administering anaesthetics or assisting the resident doctor with operations, with the proviso that care should be taken not to encroach on any established practice. The organisers hoped that having the flying doctor involved in this way would stave off boredom during periods of inactivity and compensate for professional and social isolation.

Welch reached Cloncurry to take up his post on 15 May, having travelled by air from Longreach, and was immediately thrown into the thick of it. 'On arrival there was a good crowd at the aerodrome. After a general round of introductions I was informed that Dr Shepherdson [from Cloncurry hospital] would like to speak to me privately. Shepherdson said, "Doctor, it is rather rough to ask you to come straight to the hospital, but I have a man waiting on the operating table who has cut his throat." Now the patient had been brought 50 miles by ambulance, and had lost a lot of blood on the journey – surely a case for aerial transport, if ever there was one.'[4] Welch was assisted at the operation before rejoining the official welcoming function. This was his introduction to his new duties!

The first actual flight took place on 17 May 1928 – a routine call to Julia Creek nursing home where Welch performed two minor operations. The Flying Doctor Service was officially airborne! As the first flying doctor in Australia, Welch had an important role to play. He was conscious that the future of the service would depend to a large extent on how satisfactorily he carried out the job. Taking a leaf out of Flynn's book, Welch kept various magazines appraised of his work so that the public could judge for themselves the effectiveness of the AMS and be ready to support it when the need arose. It was generally accepted that if one life was saved during that crucial first year, the benefit would be beyond question. The proof was supplied in this account from Welch who discreetly made the point that the availability of a doctor to fly in to perform an operation was instrumental in avoiding a tragedy:

> Dr Taylor, of Boulia, telephoned to me that he had a man in
> hospital, who had just been brought in 80 miles by car. He had
> diagnosed acute appendicitis and asked me to go to Boulia,
> two hundred miles south of Cloncurry. The message came at
> 2 o'clock and I saw the man at 5 pm. He was a very good type
> of stockman, and his employer, who had brought him in, told me
> that he was one of the most useful men in the district. Dr Taylor
> asked me to operate, he giving the anaesthetic. There is no need
> to go into the medical details but most folk know that a
> gangrenous appendix on the third day of illness does not usually
> prolong life. It is enough to say that the patient is doing very well
> and giving no anxiety.[5]

The romance of the Flying Doctor Service was never more apparent than in early newspaper articles chronicling its achievements with headlines such as 'Help from the Skies', 'Aid from the Air', 'I Flew with the Flying Doctor', 'Flying Doctor Brings Relief to Sufferer', 'No Rest for Flying Doctor', 'Healing Wings' and 'Doctor

Flies to Girl's Aid'. But the reality behind these somewhat fanciful descriptions was that the flying doctors, in the early years of the service, had to contend with some fairly significant problems, one of which was surely a lack of flying experience.

When the aerial medical idea was first being explored, Flynn, in a 1919 edition of *The Inlander*, made the rather extravagant claim: 'Besides the pilots ... you must have doctors *used* to the sensation of flying: mere bravery and readiness will not enable medical men to serve in this capacity. Only picked and practised doctors can experience the peculiar antics of wings, and the wobbles in balances of body air-pressures caused by necessary lightning changes of altitude, without temporarily losing their keenness of insight, and their highest delicacy of touch.'[6] Admittedly, at this point Flynn was trying to interest the defence forces in becoming involved and therefore had an ulterior motive in implying that aerial doctors would need to be trained airmen. But notwithstanding Flynn's thoughts on the matter, one can only assume that in actuality not many of the first aerial doctors would have had flying experience – and there is nothing in Flynn's writing up to that point to suggest that he had any either. Indeed, when Dr George Simpson made his first medical flight in advance of the setting up of the Cloncurry base, he confessed in a letter to his mother that the trip was 'interesting for me, but not pleasant, as I almost disgraced myself by being airsick'.[7]

Welch's successor, Dr Atcheson Spalding, also sheepishly admitted to an occasion when motion sickness inhibited his enjoyment of a flight: 'On the morning of our journey from Winton, the trip might have been described in airy terms as being rather "bumpy", and feeling a little uncertain of my inner self as time went on, I had ceased to take more than a casual interest in the endless ranges of low, brown hills, which seemed to glide beneath us.'[8] Even as late as 1937 when Jean White became the flying doctor for the Normanton base, it was reported in an article about her in the *Sydney Morning Herald* that 'when she joined the Australian Inland Mission ... she had never been up in a plane'.[9] That situation was soon addressed, as she went on to fly thousands of kilometres, undaunted even by a crash-landing in 1939 which left her and her pilot stranded for several days.

Unfamiliarity with the sensation of flying was not the only problem for the early flying doctors. They flew in aircraft devoid of the comfort and safety features of today's models and they had no sophisticated medical equipment on board for emergency procedures. If ambulance facilities were needed to transfer a critical patient to hospital on their return, they lacked the means to arrange this either from the air or from the point of pick up if there was no telephone (usually the case).

Added to these difficulties were the trials involved in reaching the sick or injured once the plane had landed. With adequate airstrips still not widespread, landings were often made at some distance from the homestead or settlement, forcing the doctor to hike through bush, travel over rough tracks sometimes on horseback, and even ford flooded creeks to reach the patient. Welch had one particularly gruelling call to an accident in the Selwyn Ranges in the north-west where an eighty-year-old man had been rolled on by his horse. His injuries included several broken bones. The plane landed 30 kilo-metres away and it was dark by the time Welch reached the patient and his companions. They were thoroughly exhausted, having carried their injured mate, a heavy man, through many kilometres of moun-tainous terrain on a makeshift stretcher to arrive at this meeting place. Welch takes up the story of their journey to a hut where they were to wait out the night: 'It was very dark. I walked ahead, leading the horses and lit spinifex bushes at intervals of about 50 yards, and this made a great blaze and lit the way. The men were so tired and sore that they could only go about a hundred yards at a time. Then they rested a few minutes and battled on again.'[10] When they finally reached the plane the following morning, it took seven people to get the patient into the machine without further damage to his broken parts. Bill 'Swampy' Marsh, referring to this event in his book *Great Flying Doctor Stories*, says that when the old man returned home after a three-month recuperation the first thing he did was go to the local pub and pass the hat around for the AMS.[11]

Over a decade later reports of hazardous exploits by flying doctors were still being reported. The facilities on board the aircraft and at the base might have improved but the nature of outback conditions, against which there was no man-made antidote, continued. In 1941 Dr John Woods from the Broken Hill base was called to attend a sick baby at Durham Downs station. The station was ringed with flood-waters and a hazardous landing was made nearby by pilot Hugh Bond. The doctor made his way to the homestead and, on his return, was forced to struggle waist-deep through mud and water holding the sick baby above his head, while the father walked alongside in case the doctor slipped. The incident ended well and the baby was flown to a nearby hospital.[12] Such incidents illustrate the justifiable acclaim given to the flying doctors' work.

Such incidents also graphically illustrate how desperately an AMS had been needed. Once established, the Cloncurry base covered a large expanse, but the rest of the outback was still outside its range. In the remainder of the Inland there were few towns of sufficient size to support a private medical practitioner. For instance, while there was a doctor at Port Augusta in South Australia and at Kalgoorlie in Western Australia, on the entire length of the transcontinental line between the two townships, a distance of a 1610 kilometres, there was no other medical centre. And it was difficult for local authorities to attract competent medical practitioners when the inducements, both profes-sionally and socially, were not great. At this time, the AIM was shouldering practically the entire nursing services of the Inland.[13]

Bruce Plowman, patrol padre for Central Australia, made a penetrating observation in 1921 about the difference between the facilities available to people in cities versus what was on offer for people of the Inland.

Of those who have the comforts and blessings of modern
civilisation, doctors, nurses, hospitals, schools, colleges, railways,

daily mails, daily newspapers, churches, Sunday Schools, etc., and
all sorts of entertainment practically at their doors, I would ask
[them] to just think of what it means to send, anywhere from
100 to 600 or 700 miles, for medical assistance of any description,
over rough, unmade tracks, fording rivers miles wide in flood
times, and over miles of soft sandhills, and through days of
sand-storms, in the heat of summer, with the glass at anywhere
between 100 and 120 in the shade, with often a slow moving
camel as the only means of transit; the same distance to the
nearest railway, and in many instances to the nearest school or
church; mails only once per fortnight or month, and in the very
back of beyond perhaps three months apart.[14]

Despite these disadvantages, outback settlers accepted their lot for
the most part with equanimity. They dealt with sickness and injury as
best they could, treating maladies with simple bush remedies like
bread for poultices or roughly cut bark for splints, or with patent
medicines, the value of which was limited despite their labels bearing
extravagant claims to the contrary. Inlanders were a hardy group, their
constitutions improved by physical work and outdoor living, if not by
a diet that consisted primarily of salt beef, damper and black tea. As
Bruce Plowman observed in his book *The Man from Oodnadatta*, the
two foods most difficult for the bushman to live without were
dripping and onions.

Without them food becomes flat and tasteless; the man on the
restricted diet of the bushman craves for them as a drunkard
craves for drink. With bread and meat the staple articles of diet,
and with long periods without fresh vegetables and milk, these
two homely varieties of food become of relatively priceless value.
Quite frequently in his travels the padre had given men two or
three onions he had carried for many miles, and had been
rewarded with gratitude altogether disproportionate to the

intrinsic value of the gift. Consequently, he carried as regularly as possible, as part of his equipment, onions as well as hymn books.[15]

A further example of the longing for that which was unattainable is wryly noted in *No Roads Go By*, written by Myrtle Rose White, covering her seven years living in the far north-east of South Australia in the early 1900s.

> There were times ... when I would have considered a lamb chop
> above rubies, cabbage food for the gods, and a beautiful scented
> rose a fair exchange for my soul.[16]

She further comments on the torment of being without fresh water.

> Rain water became so precious it had to be reserved for the
> children alone, and for the first time in my life I felt that I could
> truly sympathize with a drinker's craving. Oh, for a drink of cold,
> clear rain water! Hundreds and thousands of gallons of it run to
> waste somewhere every day! A drink of iced lemon-squash
> would be beyond price.[17]

Various problems plagued the Inlanders by very reason of their living in the outback, not least of which was the possibility of someone who was lost perishing from thirst and exposure. Arch Grant, in his book *Camel Train & Aeroplane*, mentions the case of a young medical officer and his wife who died while going to a call on the waterless track between Tennant Creek and Rockhampton Downs in the scorching summer of 1941–42. One assumes the couple were newcomers to the outback, but even experienced bushmen could find themselves in similar circumstances if, through misadventure, a trip was unexpectedly lengthened and their supplies of water became depleted. Dr George Simpson explains the range of illnesses that beset

Inlanders and the terms that were commonly used to explain them. 'Medical conditions were generally referred to as "fever" and might be anything from typhoid to malaria. Vitamin deficiency diseases are referred to as "Barcoo" when symptoms include anorexia, vomiting and debility; or "Barcoo rot" when cuts and scratches become the site of impetiginous infection. Fly-borne infection of eyes is referred to as "sandy blight" and causes much disability. Intestinal infections are not common amongst permanent residents, but newcomers and travellers rarely escape. Bore water is generally blamed.' [18]

The nature of outback work, involving farm implements, firearms, riding horses at breakneck speed, using poisons for eradicating pests, or working in industries like mining where modern safety regulations did not apply, made Inlanders prey to horrific accidents and injuries. When struck down, the bushman could usually rely on a mate to carry him whatever distance was required to seek trained help, but with doctors and hospitals few and far between, the trip itself was likely to kill him off completely or severely inhibit his chances of making a recovery. Few people had any real knowledge of first aid, a situation Flynn identified early in his career, and which he sought to address in *The Bushman's Companion*. When brought out by Flynn in 1910, this publication included basic first aid instruction about bandaging, splinting, and stemming blood flow, as well as advice on dealing with choking, poisoning and snakebite. It was prefaced by this very sound advice: 'Do practise First Aid *before trouble comes!* Make a *fad* of it in every shearing hut and splitting camp! Stopping the most dangerous bleeding in many cases is mere child's play. Then *don't let it baffle you!*' [19] Preventative medicine for people in the bush, an important part of the RFDS's current charter, was also Flynn's ideal.

Flynn himself was obliged to resort to a bushman's remedy when he was ill from the effects of the fierce heat on a trip to Central Australia in 1913. 'The situation called for desperate remedies', he wrote phlegmatically. 'After a survey of our combined larder and medicine chest I was put on a diet of dry toast, raw onions and salt.

This was followed by a draught of syrup from a tin of pineapple. Whatever the sickness was it gave up in despair'.[20] Despite his cheerful acceptance of his own situation, Flynn was nonetheless disturbed by the generally parlous state of medical and surgical facilities that he observed in his journeying around the South Australian outback. 'The people are not quite destitute. For instance, when a man gets injured near a telegraph station (you have a station every 100 miles or so along the O.T. line), you may call up a doctor in Adelaide, get his advice by wire, and take his medicine mostly by imagination.'[21] This was written four years before the dramatic operation on Jimmy Darcy that used precisely this procedure.

Nonetheless, people in the outback managed as best they could. To the question, 'What did you do before the days of the Flying Doctor?' one old-timer answered, 'You looked for the nearest sensible woman.'[22] This illustrates the tacit understanding that women in the outback were the unofficial custodians of the health of everyone around them, even if the role was not one of their choosing. City women taking up outback life through marriage to a station owner or manager underwent an abrupt transition from having the support of family and facilities to isolation and a lack of amenities. They invariably had little real experience in handling medical emergencies, but were thrown in at the deep end, learning to fight light-headedness in order to stitch wounds or splint broken limbs, or nursing family and stationhands through illnesses to which they were barely able to give a name. Even children were pressed into service when no other help was available, with the eldest girl of the family perhaps called upon to assist her mother in childbirth.

Early female settlers like Mrs Aeneas Gunn (author of *We of the Never-Never*) knew the trauma of having to assume responsibility for the care of the sick without the skills to do justice to the task. Despite fighting 'fiercely' for him, she had to watch her own husband die from malaria dysentery, nearly two decades before the establishment of a relatively nearby cottage hospital might have resulted in a different

outcome. Myrtle Rose White tells of reluctantly attending a neighbour's premature labour simply because she was the only woman
available in the area. '"There is no chance of getting her to a doctor",
says the distracted husband, "No chance of getting a doctor to her".'[23]
Newly arrived in the bush herself, Mrs White was forced to do what
she could for the stricken woman, finding reserves of courage in
herself that she had never dreamed existed. Despite her efforts, when
the bush mother was at last delivered of her child, it was stillborn.

20

Lifting the Burden

. . . .

The presence of a doctor who was readily contactable via the Flying Doctor network was of immense comfort to the nursing sisters in the various bush hospitals. The people of the bush had implicit faith in the nursing sisters' capacity to fix almost any complaint, a faith which caused them many anxious moments. Before the advent of radio, and despite being extremely well trained, the nurses nonetheless suffered agonies when they had to cope with medical emergencies that in a city hospital would automatically have been dealt with by skilled doctors or specialists. Sister Elizabeth Burchill gives this account from her time at Innamincka hostel:

> In our medical work, through sheer necessity, we learnt something of the art of diagnosis and with no wireless communication we often wondered what we could do if some surgical emergency arose. There comes to mind the case of a newcomer to Innamincka, a visiting stockman subject to attacks of abdominal pain. Our urgent problem was; is the stomach trouble caused by the appendix or not. Was it colic? The great risk of a wrongly treated or neglected appendix is peritonitis. Delay could be extremely dangerous as peritonitis is a very grave condition.

However, the stockman's stomach attacks subsided naturally, and we sent the patient 200 miles to the doctor at Tibooburra. Two days after his arrival he was operated on for appendicitis![1]

Before the appearance of the AMS, others too were obliged to render medical assistance, despite this being far beyond the scope of their usual jobs. A policeman from Anthony's Lagoon in the Gulf country explained the position:

> Speaking from my own personal viewpoint as a police officer in this part of the world, where everybody in trouble of any kind whatsoever comes of necessity to the police for assistance, the fact of the existence of the flying doctor is a very comforting one. Situated as I am here, on the junction of two great stock routes along which every year come many thousands of travelling cattle with their attendant droving plants, I am in a position to receive many sick and injured people in the year, and do so receive them. Most are received and treated by me successfully, and nobody hears of them. At times, however, comes a case with which I cannot cope, and it is then that the Flying Medical Service takes from my shoulders the responsibility such as it is, in my opinion, distinctly wrong for any layman to be called upon to bear.[2]

Outback people, enduring hardships unfamiliar to city people, were grateful recipients of the Flying Doctor Service. By the end of its first year, Welch had tended to patients over an immense distance extending to the north beyond Normanton, to the far north-west to Newcastle Waters, west to Avon Downs and south to Bedourie. The aerial medical experiment was generally regarded as fully justified, although there had been a few problems – the Flying Doctor had occasionally been called to injuries or illnesses which proved trivial, and in some cases had failed to be called in time. The latter circumstance arose partly because of the tendency of hardy citizens to endure pain and ill health without complaint and partly because the distances involved in reaching the nearest telephone or telegraph to ask for assistance were so great.

With Welch's tour of duty completed, appeals were broadcast for a replacement. According to an assessment in an article in *The Medical Journal of Australia* at the time, a doctor was needed who was experienced and resourceful, 'prepared to sacrifice a year for an ideal, ready to take risks, to endure discomfort, to forget self interests'.[3] Dr Atcheson Spalding became that man and took over the reins in May 1929. By the end of his term the AMS was firmly entrenched and was working in harmony with kindred services; local feeling was increasing in favour of the Service, local doctors were not antagonistic, and a sense of security, always high on Flynn's agenda, was being engendered among the bush people. The time seemed ripe to extend the Service but the effect of the Depression dashed any hope of sufficient funds to allow that to occur.

By the time Allan Vickers took over as flying doctor in the early 1930s, the AMS was in a precarious financial position. Vickers not only carried out his role as flying doctor with distinction, but also rendered invaluable service fundraising and generally raising the profile of the organisation via an exhaustive round of lecture tours. Vickers's name became synonymous with the Flying Doctor Service. He served in Cloncurry and later was instrumental in mustering support and giving advice in Western Australia for the setting up of bases at Wyndham and Port Hedland, modelled on Cloncurry. He became the first flying doctor at Port Hedland. During the war he joined the Australian Army Medical Corps and was put in charge of a military hospital in Western Australia. Discharged in 1943 when the threat of Japanese invasion had receded, he took up the post of flying doctor at the newly created base at Charleville in Queensland.

In 1958, Vickers, then medical superintendent of the Queensland Section, outlined the nature of the work done by the RFDS, three decades after its inception. He pointed out that although urgent flights were sometimes made in unusual circumstances, attracting spectacular press coverage, most flights were routine. Doctors attended to the same range of illnesses and injuries, both minor and major, as did their city counterparts. In addition, they conducted routine visits at regular intervals to isolated communities and bush hospitals. They cooperated in the various state poliomyelitis campaigns during which thousands of children received the Salk vaccine. Advice by radio was given, enabling mothers in isolated areas to cope with minor ailments. Vickers said in his article: 'Please do not sniff superiorly at the idea of diagnosis and treatment by radio. This is a field in which one can improve tremendously by practice. It is fascinating to find how accurate the diagnosis can become by the use of the doctor's trained mind and the bush-dweller's eyes and fingers, coordinated by several hundred miles of radio communication. It is good training in systematic, orderly diagnostic thinking.'[4]

Not only could doctors diagnose by remote control, they could also give instructions as to how a patient might be helped by those around them without a flight being necessary. A published account of a medical drama, reported in Elizabeth Burchill's book *Innamincka*, illustrates how the flying doctor, from the base, was able to instruct a nursing sister on a rather grisly procedure:

> In a chair by the wireless set at the Nursing Home sat a grim-faced man with a dislocated shoulder. By his side stood the police officer of the Innamincka district, a stockman and the mission Sister. With the operator at Broken Hill acting as intermediary, the doctor from his own study gave instructions, while the Sister pedalled for dear life, and the two hefty male 'nurses' carried out instructions which she threw over her shoulder from her position at the set.
>
> 'Hold his elbow close to his side. Have you got that? Over to you.'
>
> 'We are holding his elbow close to his side. What next? Over to you.'

And so it went on until a grunt from the patient and a dull click from the shoulder caused a delighted Sister to exclaim: 'Got it! It's clicked in!' And the flying doctor network had made history again.[5]

An important part of the successful development of diagnosis by radio or phone was the introduction of medical chests for use at outposts, and the famous body chart. In 1939 Dr Keith Sweetman, the flying doctor for Wyndham in Western Australia, suggested supplying standardised medical chests to enable the layperson to carry out home treatment at the direction of the flying doctor at the base. This idea was further developed by a sub-committee involving doctors George Simpson and Allan Vickers. The chest would include all the drugs, medicines, instruments and equipment (such as bandages and dressings) for treatment of the most commonly diagnosed illnesses and complaints. It was a lockable steel chest with a series of shelves containing the various medications. Each was numbered so that there would be no confusion when the doctor recommended a particular medicine and gave instruction regarding its use. 'Give Tommy one tablet of number four every four hours, and a teaspoonful of number twenty-six after each meal and let me know tomorrow how he is.'[6] The chest cost twelve pounds. Also included was a simple anatomical chart. This was the brainchild of nursing sister Lucy Garlick from Broome in Western Australia. The chart showed a human body, front and back, with each section of the body numbered. This was a great help in long-range diagnosis, enabling the patient to describe the part of the body in pain by simply nominating a numbered area. These charts still exist in the modern medical chests, although many doctors no longer rely on them, preferring instead to use their own words to tell the patient what to feel for and where.

Dr W Scott Kennedy, flying doctor at Broken Hill in the late 1940s, outlines the problems inherent in radio diagnosis before a large audience: 'My first radio session was rather confusing, although I must say that the folk at the other end were very patient and helpful. How does one go about asking personal questions when there are probably a few hundred other folk listening? How do you ask a single girl if she is pregnant? You resort to a lot of circumlocution, but eventually you may have to ask the direct question. Making a diagnosis under these circumstances is very difficult.'[7]

A further amusing anecdote from Dr Kennedy concerns the use of medical chests. He writes:

> The owner of a station, who was one of our most frequent customers, had about six children and had sent us a photograph of them all lined up and numbered one to six. When asking advice he would refer to the particular chid by number. This day he got on the radio, 'Hey doc, number four has a cough and is spitting up phlegm – he isn't hot. Number two has cut his foot' and so on through the tribe. I prescribed from the medical chest suitable treatment. The whole point of the story is that having prescribed an expectorant cough mixture for number four and finished the medical session, I sat back and listened to the radiograms. What did I hear? Our friend ordering from the grocer, amongst other items, six bottles of Heenzo, a cure-all for chest and throat troubles, and sold by grocers.[8]

The medical chests, with some additions and omissions to the original set-up, are still a vital component of health care for remote areas. The Commonwealth Department of Health and Ageing funds the supply and replenishment of approximately 3000 of these medical chests scattered throughout outback Australia, at pastoral properties, outstations, Indigenous communities, remote mining sites, police stations, and with travelling field parties. Periodically the contents are reviewed to ensure the relevancy and currency of pharmaceuticals. Users take responsibility for keeping their chests up to date and replenished, but more recently computerised chest management systems have been incorporated by various sections.

In the early days pilots were loath to fly at night with no instruments to guide them through the darkness and no established system of lighting at landing strips, so doctors were forced to perform emergency operations in primitive circumstances if the urgency of a case precluded waiting for a daylight take-off. Pilots were sometimes involved more intimately in such medical procedures than they might have chosen to be. Harry Hudson, in *Flynn's Flying Doctors*, records an interview with Dr Allan Vickers, then based at Charleville. Vickers had been called to a patient who needed an emergency operation. This was performed on the kitchen table, with pilot Ron Anderson taking the role of anaesthetist. Although a little pale throughout the ordeal, the pilot struggled on gamely and carried out his temporary assignment without complaint.[9] Nowadays, the flight nurse would be on hand for tasks like these, but aircraft flying speeds are such that it is rare for a patient not to be transferred to the nearest hospital for emergency operations. Nonetheless, certain procedures and interventions are often necessary to stabilise a patient's condition pre-flight and these may have to be carried out in less than ideal working conditions.

Allan Vickers features prominently in the RFDS story because of the longevity of his service but others, too, were well known for particular reasons. One was Dr Harold Dicks who was a huge figure in the Western Australia Section because of the multiple roles he carried out – doctor, pilot, aircraft maintenance engineer and administrator. He took over at Port Hedland when Allan Vickers was transferred to the army hospital in Perth and began a decades-long association with the RFDS. His operation was moved inland to Marble Bar when it was considered that the coast was vulnerable to further attacks from Japanese bombers. Adding to his notoriety in the early 1970s his wife Robin Miller was also employed by the RFDS as a pilot and, as a triple-certificated nurse, occasionally stepped into flight nurse mode for her husband. Dicks further served the RFDS by flying newly purchased aircraft from America back to Australia for the use of the service. On many of these flights, Robin Miller flew as co-pilot.

Another well-known personality in RFDS history was Irish-born Timothy O'Leary, a doctor employed by the Queensland Section in 1953, who served at all its operational bases. He also followed in the steps of Allan Vickers and served as chief medical officer in Brisbane. Once ensconced as flying doctor at Charters Towers, he sent for his Irish fiancée and they were married that year. Tragically, while accompanying her husband on a routine flight six weeks later, their plane crashed and Catherine O'Leary was killed, along with the pilot Captain Martin Garrett. (Captain Garrett's wife Beth joined the RFDS in the Queensland Section in 1968. She was its first woman pilot, and when she retired twenty years later in 1988, the longest-serving.)

Dr O'Leary's distinctive personality, medical skills and knowledge of aircraft (he held a private pilot's licence) earned him a considerable reputation during the twenty-seven years he served with the Queensland Section. He retired in 1980. He wrote two fascinating books recording his many adventures, both medical and aerial, involving himself, his pilots and other doctors. One spine-tingling story concerned a search and rescue mission that O'Leary undertook to locate Dr Ewart Smith and pilot Cliff Parsons from Cloncurry who had crash-landed on a claypan in the Gulf area. O'Leary's pilot negotiated a tricky landing at a distance from the stricken plane but the rescue still had a way to go because between the two aircraft was a watercourse infested with crocodiles. During the preceding night the stranded men had sought refuge from these predators in the cabin of the plane, the crocodiles' footprints around the claypan in the morning attesting to the wisdom of this decision. Smith then resolved to make a dash for the rescue aircraft and O'Leary's pilot fired a couple of rounds from a rifle to clear the path. No ripples appeared in the water, indicating the absence, however temporary, of crocodiles.

Wrote O'Leary: 'This was enough evidence for the doctor. He took off at full speed down the sloping bank and made a spectacular running dive. From the moment he hit the water, all we could see was a churning maelstrom advancing towards us. He landed without incident, a very relieved and happy man.'[10] The pilot, not a strong swimmer, decided that discretion was the better part of valour and elected to stay with the plane until a land rescue party arrived.

21

The Modern Approach

. . . .

Seventy-five years after its inception, the RFDS still provides the basic ministration that John Flynn envisaged for it at the outset, but today there are many more facilities and services offered. As outlined in the *2002 Annual Report*, the role of the Flying Doctor Service is comprehensive, including 24-hour emergency services, primary health care clinics at remote sites, female GP clinics, telephone consultations and inter-hospital transfers.[1] In the year 2001/2002, the service attended to 196 996 patients and carried out 25 977 aerial evacuations. There were 8861 health care clinics conducted and 57 085 telehealth consultations (mainly by telephone with a small number by radio).[2] Operating from twenty-one locations across Australia, there is no other organisation in the world that provides a similar range of services over such an immense, yet sparsely populated, area and in such a variety of climatic conditions. Flying Doctor territory ranges from places just one hour out of most of Australia's capital cities to the most far-flung reaches of the continent.

The emergency health services, with which the RFDS is most commonly associated, are provided around the clock – every day of the year – to care for victims of illness or accident who are in serious or potentially life-threatening situations. Despite the importance of this activity, however, it represents only a small portion of the total service provided by the RFDS for people in rural and remote Australia. Nonetheless, emergency cases take priority over all else. Once the call for help has been received, pilot, doctor and flight nurse, with precision borne of practice, can be airborne within a very short space of time.

When an emergency call is received, the doctor rostered for emergency duty carries out a medical assessment and assigns a priority: priority 1 – the situation is considered life-threatening and the team will be on its way within thirty to forty-five minutes; priority 2 – not life-threatening, but evacuation required as soon as possible; and priority 3 – non-urgent, evacuation will be undertaken when resources are available.[3] This system allows flight crew to gauge how quickly they will need to be on their way and enables personnel to determine, if there are two competing cases, which will be dealt with first. As Senior Medical Officer Dr Mike Hill puts it:

'Sometimes, you have to work out what you need to respond to
right now and, in the meantime, while you're dealing with one,
is there another way of dealing with the other? Is it possible for
a nurse to get out to see them? Is it possible by some other means
to get access to care in the meantime? The difficult part of the
job is always the logistics. The easy part is the medicine. You
know what treatment they need – what assessment they need.
The difficulty is making it all happen.'

Doctors called to an emergency situation prefer to perform all their medical procedures before loading the patient onto the plane to avoid having to work in the cramped environment of the aircraft. In these situations they have to tread a delicate path between doing too little and endangering the patient, or doing too much, and unnecessarily lengthening the time before the patient is admitted to a hospital. According to Mike Hill, the skill lies in doctors knowing where to draw the line and knowing when to say, 'OK I've done enough – let's go'. He points out that there are sometimes logistical problems outside their control that increase time at the scene when they are trying to keep it down. In rare instances emergency procedures may carry the event into night-time on a strip unsuitable for take-off out of daylight hours and the patient then has to be transported to the nearest night strip. These are the difficulties that the flying doctor grapples with on a daily basis. In addition they have to be prepared to deal with an enormous variety of medical conditions. Senior Medical Officer Dr Don Bowley says that the type of cases covered by flying doctors cover the complete range, from patients who are critically ill with heart disease, emphysema, asthma, renal disease, liver disease, appendicitis, cholecystitis, to any sort of major trauma due to car accidents, bike accidents, falls from horses and injuries due to violence like stabbings, bashings, and shootings.

While medical personnel stand by for these emergencies, RFDS doctors, nurses and other specialised health professionals conduct a network of primary health care clinics at isolated sites – Aboriginal and Torres Strait Islander communities, remote stations, mines and oilfields, rural support towns, national parks and island resorts. These services include but are not limited to routine health checks and advice, immunisation, child health care, dental, eye and ear clinics.[4] Patients who present at the clinics with a more significant injury or illness that can't be managed locally are evacuated to the nearest hospital. Most of the clinics are conducted in townships which have a small primary health centre staffed by nurses or health workers. This might be a purpose-built building or simply the local hall pressed into service. Other locations in which the medical staff conduct their clinics can include a room in a station homestead, an outstation or mine site, in the plane itself or on the ground in the shade of a wing tip.

In some areas of the far west where smaller towns are in decline and losing GPs, the Flying Doctor has stepped into the breach to provide GP services. Flying doctors have compensated for doctor shortages at other points too in history, particularly during the Second World War, when flying doctors attended townships whose medical partitioners had enlisted in the services.

One constant for the Service is the provision of consultations by doctors connected to their patients at remote locations by telephone or, less frequently in modern times, by radio. In these instances, the doctor is like an ordinary GP. They get to know their patients and their medical histories and provide advice in the same way as a city GP does. The essential difference is that they do not actually see the person who calls for help. In fact, country people boast that they can contact the Flying Doctor for a consultation more quickly than the average city dweller who has to make an appointment and travel the necessary distance to a surgery. With a physical examination not possible, the doctor depends on the patient or carer to describe the symptoms accurately, a situation made easier if the patient is at a rural clinic and a health worker can provide the hands and eyes. Dr Don Bowley explains:

> Initially there is a rapid learning curve. After a while you get
> more comfortable with it but you're only as good as the
> information you're given. The skill is in making sure that you
> have the information you need to make a reliable phone
> diagnosis. There is a degree of educated guessing. The rural and
> remote nurses are very good and give you reliable information
> and can examine the patient to gain further insight. The
> challenge is in the more remote locations where the person on
> the phone does not have much medical knowledge or
> experience. Fortunately most outback people have a lot of
> common sense. However, some people don't want to trouble you
> or they underestimate what is wrong with them – it's only a bit
> of a cut and you get there and there's a massive laceration going
> down half the leg. Other people overestimate what is wrong with

them – they're practically dying and you get there and they don't have a lot wrong with them. If you've been in the job for a fair while you usually know most of the people – you've talked to them many times on the phone. You know who gets a bit excited and who doesn't. You get a feeling for the people.

The doctor may recommend some medication from the medical chest and give advice on how to take it and how often, then keep in constant touch to monitor progress. If the patient fails to improve, the doctor will make the decision to fly out and examine the patient in person. In bases like Broken Hill, clients visiting the township for shopping or business appointments might consult with a doctor at the base, always accepting that the doctor of their choice may be called out suddenly to attend an emergency situation.

The Service is also on hand to transfer patients to large metropolitan hospitals from smaller rural and remote area hospitals which lack facilities for specialised medical procedures.

When John Flynn set up his network of cottage hospitals in the Inland staffed by well-qualified sisters, he was attempting to improve the well-being of all Inlanders by giving them access to some form of health care at least reasonably close at hand. In particular, though, he recognised the specific need for women to have the security of such medical facilities in order to encourage them to go to the outback, and once there, to stay and bring up their families in relative safety. This concept is not dissimilar to the thinking behind the establishment of the Rural Women's GP Program begun in 2000. The program is funded by the Commonwealth Government, with the RFDS acting as the facilitating body to coordinate the delivery of female GPs to rural and remote locations of all states and the Northern Territory. The program recognises the right of these women to have the health care of their choice in the same way that their city cousins do. Female GPs attend these identified rural communities where there is little or no access to female practitioners and deliver a range of services including cervical screening and breast examination. The majority of Rural Women GP Program clinics are conducted in existing local GP practices which ensures continuity of care and detailed insight into the cultural diversity of the local community. For indigenous women and for women from ethnic backgrounds, the availability of a female doctor can be especially important. During the 2001/2002 financial year there were 612 clinics conducted at the ninety-eight sites throughout Australia which resulted in 8897 consultations.[5] The success of this service has resulted in plans for additional clinics of this type in the future.

The RFDS has developed other initiatives over the years in response to the demonstrated needs of people in the bush, chief of which was its national strategic plan 'The Best for the Bush' published in 1993 and designed as a guide to future directions for the RFDS. Apart from recommendations to maintain and refine the well-established emergency services of the RFDS, major new initiatives were proposed in the area of non-emergency services. Areas identified as possibilities for future development were health promotion, Aboriginal and Torres Strait Islander health, mental health, women's health, and child and adolescent health.

A priority concern was the issue of mental health. While RFDS doctors and nurses have always been mindful of the part that mental health plays in good physical health, it has often been done quite informally by providing a sympathetic ear when the need arose, a huge boon to people who sometimes allow their much-vaunted country stoicism to prevent them from complaining.

This has been the case ever since Flynn first began to champion the cause of people in the bush. A comment was published in *The Inlander* in 1929 under the heading 'A Woman's Point of View' at a time when the nursing sisters in the cottage hospitals were still bearing most of the burden of providing social welfare for the Inlanders, and says in part: 'Sometimes, if you are not sick in body, you are sick in mind, and even just to know that the hospital is there means much to lonely men and women. If you can drop in and have a talk, and have somebody else's cakes and scones, with a new book under your arm, and some new thoughts in your mind – you feel a different being.'[6] As things change so they stay the same.

Mental health took on a more formal aspect for the RFDS with a study in 1995 that confirmed the presence of mental health issues in the bush and looked at the feasibility of providing a service to address these issues in conjunction with the RFDS. It was acknowledged that people in the bush had the same reasons for depression as people elsewhere – alcohol and drug addiction, family break-ups, domestic violence, financial difficulties and the grim spectre of a rising rate of suicide. Added to these is the psychological strain placed on rural families by economic decline, shrinking populations, contracting services and social isolation, and more recently, the destructive nature of drought conditions causing outback people to question whether they will be able to stay with their businesses and properties or be forced to give up a lifetime's work and walk away.

An example of the attempt to redress these problems was the commencement of a three-year mental health program in the Queensland Section begun in 1996 following a one-year feasibility study. The program included such initiatives as the appointment of a psychologist operating from the Cairns base to service communities in its catchment area and was extended in 2000 to include an additional psychologist.

Psychologists are part of the primary health care side of the Service and join the regular clinic runs together with the doctor who does a general practice clinic and the nurse who does a child health clinic. They run a psychology clinic and see patients either referred by an RFDS doctor or nurse, or by a remote area nurse.

Cairns-based Robert Williams, the first of the psychologists to be employed by the RFDS, says that there has been some resistance to the program mainly because of the stigma attached to mental health problems, strong everywhere but quite noticeable in the bush. He explains: 'Self reliance and stoicism are highly valued in the bush and that delays people, particularly men, seeking help.' The stigma is overcome by the psychologist seeing people and helping people and the small communities then seeing the benefit. Also crucial to the acceptance of the program is in linking it to the RFDS, an organisation with existing bush credibility. Robert goes on: 'My approach and the approach of our current psychologist is to take a very pragmatic practical approach, not an airy fairy lying-on-the-couch type approach. We tackle it in a way which I think is better accepted. We often sit under a tree or lean over a fence and talk through with people how they can practically overcome a situation.'

An important addendum to the mental health program has been the development of a CD-ROM, entitled 'Psychological First Aid Kit', designed as a training resource for health professionals. The CD-ROM covers the most commonly occurring mental health problems in remote communities and, via various fictional scenarios, instructs users in how to deal with them. Released in 1999, it has since been disseminated widely across Australia, particularly among RFDS staff. It is part of the organisation's commitment to educating health service providers to better detect, manage and refer mental health problems.

Because of the unique nature of the work they do, flying doctors need particular personal and medical skills. They must work effectively as part of a multi-disciplinary team. They have to be good communicators since much of their work is done by phone, and they must be skilled at interpreting what they hear without the advantage of being able to draw conclusions from a patient's facial expressions. Above all, they must be extremely quick-thinking and flexible. Theirs is not a nine-to-five job. Hours are long and irregular and their day can progress in a disjointed manner, requiring them, when the need arises, to switch quickly from an uncomplicated phone consultation for a sore throat to an emergency medical flight needing immediate action.

Doctors first joining the service are on a steep learning curve – learning to diagnose over the phone, learning to assess when to fly and when not to. They have to be mindful of the expense to the Service of making a flight weighed against the dreadful repercussions if a flight is not taken in a critical situation. It is generally acknowledged that doctors first joining the service tend to fly more, erring on the side of caution, being unwilling to run the risk of jeopardising the welfare of their patients.

Flying doctors have to be willing to make judgments regarding their patients without the diagnostic support or pathology backup present in a hospital setting. Without those aids, the challenge for the doctor called to a remote location is to have the confidence to clinically determine what's happening based only on history and physical examination.

Doctors need experience in critical and emergency care and in obstetrics, disciplines not always the province of an urban GP. Babies eager to enter the world have scant regard for time or place and there have been occasions when babies have been delivered while the plane was airborne. Bill Marsh, in *Great Flying Doctor Stories*, tells of a pilot registering the POB (persons on board) with flight control before take-off, then calling back mid-flight to request an adjustment in order to register the new arrival.[7] A similar but even more dramatic story comes from Robin Miller, a pilot and nurse who flew for the Western Australia Section in the 1970s. When travelling alone with a pregnant girl who went into unexpected labour, Miller was forced to put the plane on autopilot and deliver the baby herself. Miller's message to control, recounted in her book *Flying Nurse* was: "'Port Hedland – Foxtrot Delta Papa. Was abeam Hillside Mine, one six, six five zero zero feet, Hedland four seven. Sorry for the delay. Persons on board now increased to three." There was a short silence, then came the reply. "Congratulations, Foxtrot Delta Papa! Boy or girl?'"[8]

Doctors, flight nurses and clinic nurses have to work in conditions that can be physically trying. Not only are the facilities at clinics not as sophisticated as those in the city, but they have to battle with debilitating heat in summer (temperatures in a plane's cabin can soar when it is stationary on an outback strip), and with flies, dust and bad weather when they're working in the open. Their ride to work will often be more fraught than for an urban dweller when they are flying in poor conditions. The plane is narrow and cramped with limited headroom which makes access to the patient difficult. When noise and vibration are added to the mix, the plane, while being extremely well equipped for the purpose it fulfils, is not the most comfortable working environment. This is the downside. The upside is that doctors and nurses continue to be drawn to the Service, enticed by the professional challenges and the variety of the work – and maybe even by the romance of the Flying Doctor idea and its proud history of service.

Recruiting medical staff to the bush, however, is often difficult. The RFDS is aware of the need to provide excellent accommodation and other benefits in order to encourage medical staff to serve in these areas. Chief Medical Officer Dr Anne Wakatama explains: 'If conditions in which people have to work are too onerous they won't come to a remote area. We provide generous provisions for study leave, annual leave and time in lieu. If you don't provide people with adequate time off and reasonable fringe benefits you're not going to retain staff.'

Despite the longevity of its operation, the RFDS still has a magical attraction. To attend an RFDS open day is to witness its allure – young children peering inquisitively into the cabin of the demonstration plane and marvelling at the equipment, an elderly gentleman (himself perhaps a former airman) deep in conversation about navigational aids with a pilot, a middle-aged woman listening intently to a flight nurse and murmuring wistfully, 'If I was twenty years younger, I'd be doing this too'.

The Flying Doctor Service is about cooperation – between the people in the air and the people on the ground – when plans have to be changed suddenly and everyone has to smoothly adjust to the new circumstances. This story from an RFDS patient in 2001 illustrates:

As the dust settled and I wheezed air into my winded lungs, I saw the headless emu. Suddenly, I realised how lucky I was to be alive.

My four wheeler was zipping back from Teryawynia Lake. When I spotted the rampaging emu it was too late to do anything but hope for the best. It crashed into my buggy's steering column, ripping the handles from my hands. The force catapulted me over the handlebars and I thudded to earth 20 metres down the rough track. At least I only felt as bad as the old bird looked. Decapitated and missing a few feathers he really had come off second best.

My friends got me back to the Teryawynia homestead and called the Flying Doctor.

Although I only felt a bit shaken and sore, Broken Hill Base's Dr Lyall said he would fly out and make absolutely sure there were no spinal or head injuries.

There are a lot of trees and buildings around Teryawynia's airstrip so it can be dangerous to land a plane as large as a King Air. So the Flying Doctor used their local knowledge to find a larger strip nearby.

Glen Albyn Station an hour up the road was the only suitable place.

Flat on my back on a mattress in a ute's tray, it was 60 slow and bumpy minutes to Glen Albyn. The strip was the best of a bad bunch. With the light fading, the pilot was worried if the aircraft could accelerate and climb high enough to cover the trees and buildings. He paced out the strip and carefully did the sums.

He said he would give it a go but warned if he wasn't happy with the visibility or couldn't get enough acceleration he would abort.

With ute headlights illuminating the runway, the engines surged and we rocketed down the strip. The pilot's plan worked and we were safely airborne. After about 35 minutes, we landed in Griffith, near my home town of Coleambally, where I was taken to hospital for more tests.

Thankfully, my prognosis is much better than the emu's. I have made a good recovery and the only thing carrying any scars is my helmet.[9]

Some people enter the ranks of the RFDS, do their job, and move on. But for the majority, working for the RFDS is a more than a job – it is a vocation. They are staunchly committed to its ideals and carry out their roles with dedication and conviction. Marie Osborn, the first flying sister for the Western Australia Section, offered an opinion of her job which perhaps sums up the sentiments of many others. When asked to describe her time with the Flying Doctor Service, she said: 'I thought afterwards it was like being on top of a mountain. Once you've been up there … it's hard to be ordinary again.'[10]

This book salutes the extraordinary seventy-five-year history of the RFDS and the extraordinary people who contributed to its creation and continue to carry on its work.

Notes

. . . .

1   The Man and the Mission

1   *The Inlander*, vol. 6, no. 1, 1920, p. 38.
2   *Frontier News*, vol. 37, 1952, p. 2.
3   W Scott McPheat, *John Flynn: Apostle to the Inland*, Hodder & Stoughton, London, 1963, p. 43.
4   John Flynn, 'Introduction', in *The Bushman's Companion: A Handful of Hints for Outbackers*, Home Mission Committee of the Presbyterian Church of Victoria, Melbourne, 1910.
5   ibid, pp. 49, 50, 51, 56.
6   ibid, p. 6.
7   ibid, p. 7.
8   *The Inlander*, vol. 1, no. 1, 1913, p. 24.
9   ibid, vol. 1, no. 2, 1914, pp. 61–2.

2   The Kirk at Work

1   *The Inlander*, vol. 1, no. 3, 1914, p. 91.
2   ibid, vol. 1, no. 2, 1914, p. 92.
3   Mrs Aeneas Gunn, *We of the Never-Never*, Angus & Robertson, North Ryde, 1905, p. 4.
4   RB Plowman, *The Boundary Rider*, Angus & Robertson Ltd, Sydney, 1935, p. 123.
5   McPheat, pp. 40–1.
6   John Flynn, *Northern Territory and Central Australia: A Call to the Church*, Angus & Robertson, Sydney, 1912, p. 9.
7   ibid, p. 46.
8   McPheat, p. 74.
9   RB Plowman, *The Man from Oodnadatta*, Angus & Robertson Ltd, Sydney, 1934, p. 65.
10 *The Inlander*, vol. 1, no. 3, 1914, p. 147.
11 ibid, vol. 1, no. 1, 1913, p. 6.

12 ibid, vol. 1, no. 1, 1913, p. 12.
13 ibid, vol. 1, no. 1, 1913, p. 7.
14 ibid, vol. 1, no. 1, 1913, p. 22.

3 A Voice for the Outback

1 *The Inlander*, vol. 1, no. 3, 1914, p. 121.
2 *The Messenger*, 1919, p. 512.
3 *The Inlander*, vol. 2, no. 2, 1915, p. 55.
4 ibid, vol. 1, no. 3, 1914, p. 140.
5 ibid, vol. 1, no. 1, 1913, p. 23.
6 ibid, vol. 3, no. 1, 1916, p. 40.
7 McPheat, p. 90.
8 *The Inlander*, vol. 5, no. 1, 1918, p. 30.
9 ibid, vol. 5, no. 2, 1918–19, p. 101.

4 The Tyranny of Distance

1 *The Medical Journal of Australia*, 18 April 1959, p. 550.
2 *Early Days*, vol. 9, part 5, p. 96.
3 *The Inlander*, vol. 5, no. 1, 1918, pp. 7–10.
4 Address by Dr George Simpson, St Andrews Presbyterian Church, Gisborne, 20 April 1958.
5 *The Messenger*, 1919, p. 48.
6 ibid, p. 576.
7 *The Inlander*, vol. 6, no. 1, 1920, p. 38.
8 ibid, vol. 4, no. 2, 1917–18, p. 81.
9 ibid, vol. 5, no. 1, 1918, p. 16.

5 The Elimination of Dread

1 *The Inlander*, vol. 5, no. 2, 1918–19, p. 75.
2 McPheat, p. 96.
3 *The Inlander*, vol. 6, no. 1, 1920, pp. 36, 38.
4 ibid, vol. 6, no. 2, 1920–21, p. 79.
5 ibid, vol. 6, no. 2, 1920–21, p. 76.
6 ibid, vol. 6, no. 2, 1920–21, p. 78.
7 ibid, vol. 7, no. 1, 1922, p. 17.
8 ibid, vol. 7, no. 1, 1922, p. 21.
9 *Melbourne Herald*, 2 September 1926.
10 Ernestine Hill, *Flying Doctor Calling*, Angus & Robertson, Sydney, 1947, pp. 47–8.
11 *The Inlander*, vol. 20, 1929, p. 47.
12 AIM pamphlet, 'Report of the AIM Board', September 1928, p. 13.

6 An Aerial Medical Experiment

1 Address by Dr George Simpson, St Andrews Presbyterian Church, Gisborne, 20 April 1958.
2 George Simpson, *Diary Letters of George Simpson: June, July, August 1927*, Australian Inland Mission, 1933, p. 21.

3 ibid, p. 48.
4 Letter from Cloncurry, Rev. Andrew Barber, 7 August 1927.
5 *The Inlander*, vol. 19, 1927, p. 60.
6 AIM pamphlet, 'Aerial Medical Service', 1928.
7 *The Inlander*, vol. 20, 1929, pp. 51–2.

7 A National Movement

1 Graeme Aplin, SG Foster, & Michael McKernan (eds), *Australians: A Historical Dictionary*, Fairfax, Syme & Weldon Associates, Broadway, NSW, 1987, pp. 116–17.
2 *The Presbyterian Messenger*, 1927, p. 201.
3 *Frontier News*, vol. 67, 1967, p. 6. Used with permission of Frontier Services.
4 ibid, vol. 7, 1934, p. 3.
5 ibid, vol. 7, 1934, p. 4.
6 ibid, vol. 25, 1941, p. 13.
7 Norma King, *Wings Over the Goldfields: The 50 Year History of the Eastern Goldfields Section of the RFDS of Australia*, RFDS (Eastern Goldfields Section) and Hesperian Press, Carlisle, WA, 1992, p. 28.
8 Harry Hudson, *Flynn's Flying Doctors*, The Specialty Press Ltd, Melbourne, 1956, p. 181.
9 Hill, p. 143.
10 *Frontier News*, vol. 17, 1936, p. 3.
11 Maisie McKenzie, *Flynn's Last Camp*, Boolarong Publications, Brisbane, 1985, p. 15.
12 'Sacred Stones' from *About Us* series, SBS, 12 July 2002.
13 Simpson, p. 27.
14 *The Inlander*, vol. 6, no. 1, 1920, pp. 37–8.

8 Sending and Receiving

1 *The Inlander*, vol. 19, 1927, p. 79.
2 John Flynn, 'Bush wireless', reprinted in *Wireless Weekly*, 4 February 1927.
3 *The Inlander*, vol. 19, 1927, p. 79.
4 Michael Page, *The Flying Doctor Story 1928–1978*, Rigby, Adelaide, 1977, p. 54.
5 Fred McKay, *Traeger: The Pedal Radio Man*, Boolarong Press, Moorooka, Qld, 1995, p. 2.
6 *The Inlander*, vol. 19, 1927, p. 82.
7 ibid, p. 83.
8 McPheat, p. 148.
9 *The Inlander*, vol. 19, 1927, p. 77.

9 Pedal Power

1 *The NSW Presbyterian*, 1929, p. 734.
2 John Bilton, *The Royal Flying Doctor Service of Australia: Its Origin, Growth and Development*, Royal Flying Doctor Service of Australia, Federal Council, Sydney, 1961, p. 14.
3 *Frontier News*, vol. 25, 1941, p. 12.
4 McKay, p. 31.
5 *The NSW Presbyterian*, 1929, p. 782.
6 ibid, 1930, p. 158.
7 3AR broadcast by Dr George Simpson, 20 October 1929, published in *The Presbyterian Messenger*, 1 November 1929.

8   ibid.
9   *The NSW Presbyterian*, 1929, p. 270.
10 Hudson, p. 179.
11 *The Presbyterian Messenger*, 1929, p. 48.
12 *The NSW Presbyterian*, 1930, p. 126.
13 Elizabeth Burchill, *Innamincka*, Rigby, Adelaide, 1960, p. 115.

10   The Inland Speaks

1   Burchill, p. 116.
2   Plowman, *The Man from Oodnadatta*, p. 269.
3   *Frontier News*, vol. 4, 1932, p. 56.
4   ibid, vol. 17, 1936, p. 3.
5   *The NSW Presbyterian*, 1950, p. 11.
6   Hill, pp. 100–1.
7   *The Flying Doctor* (WA Section), Autumn 2000.
8   Hill, p. 115.
9   Transcript of a talk given to RWAHS, 18 May 1983, by Mrs LL Miller (Edith M. Miller); published in *Early Days*, vol. 9, no. 1, 1983, p. 57. Quoted by permission of Edith M Miller's daughter and executor, Patricia Grimoldby.

11   The Wireless Network in Action

1   McKay, p. 74.
2   Address for the Wireless Institute of Australia by Major General Michael Jeffery, September 1998. Published in *Amateur Radio Magazine*, September 1998.
3   *The Age*, 24 November 1950, p. 2.
4   *The Flying Doctor*, 1 October 1943, p. 51.
5   ibid, 1 July 1943, p. 46.
6   ibid, 1 July 1945, p. 57.
7   *Frontier News*, vol. 29, 1944, pp. 7–8.
8   Page, p. 110.
9   King, pp. 31–2.
10 Hudson, p. 216.
11 *The NSW Presbyterian*, 1945, p. 12.
12 Archives of the Broken Hill base of the RFDS.
13 Letter from Mrs D Forsyth, in *Frontier News*, vol. 91, no. 2, 1989, p. 11. Used with permission of Frontier Services.
14 *The Introduction of the Single Sideband System to the RFDS* booklet, January 1973.
15 Royal Flying Doctor Service website <http://www.rfds.org.au>.
16 *Royal Flying Doctor Service Annual Report 2001*, p. 3.

12   Aerial Antics

1   'History of the RFDS', in *Australian Council of the RFDS Annual Report 2002*, p. 4.
2   Page, p. 258.
3   Norman Brearley, *Australian Aviator*, Rigby, Adelaide, 1971, p. 69.

4   *The Inlander*, vol. 5, no. 1, 1918, p. 14.

5   Address by Dr George Simpson, Skipton, Victoria, 13 November 1927.

6   *The Inlander*, vol. 6, no. 2, 1920–21, p. 80.

7   Queensland & Northern Territory Aerial Services pamphlet 'A Suitable Landing Ground and How to Receive an Aeroplane', from the Qantas Founders Outback Museum.

8   Hudson Fysh, *Qantas Rising*, Angus & Robertson, Sydney, 1965, p. 150.

9   *The Flying Doctor* (NSW Section), 1 October 1943, pp. 54–5.

10 Arthur H Affleck, *The Wandering Years*, Longmans, Green, Croydon, Vic., 1964, p. 65.

11 *The Flying Doctor* (WA Section), Spring 1999.

12 *The Flying Doctor* (NSW Section), 1 July 1946, p. 1.

13 Landing and Take-off

1   Robin Miller, *Sugarbird Lady*, comp. & ed. Harold Dicks, Rigby, Adelaide, 1979, p. 45.

2   Fysh, p. 206.

3   Affleck, p. 57.

4   Fysh, p. 208.

5   *The Courier-Mail*, 1 February 1939, p. 1.

6   *The Presbyterian Messenger*, 1929, p. 672.

7   Royal Flying Doctor Service (Queensland Section) website
    <http://www.flyingdoctorqueensland.net/>

8   George Farwell, *Down Argent Street: The Story of Broken Hill*, FH Johnston Publishing, Sydney, 1948, pp. 105–9.

9   King, p. 131.

14 Airshow

1   Fysh, p. 208.

2   *Wings Over the Kimberleys*, booklet of the Flying Doctor Service of Australia (Victorian Section), 1947.

3   Letter to author from Dr W Scott Kennedy, 23 January 2003.

4   ibid.

5   Bilton, pp. 87–8.

6   Page, p. 187.

7   '30 Good Years', in *The Flying Doctor* (WA Section), Spring, 1999, p. 22.

8   *RFDS of Australia Federal Council Annual Report 1983*, p. 5.

9   Royal Flying Doctor Service, Federal Council, *Royal Flying Doctor Service of Australia: Australia's Unique Outback Medical Organisation*, Sydney, 1990, p. 544.

10 Robert B Cooter, *The Air Doctors of South Australia: A Brief History of Medicine in Aero-Medical Operations in South Australia, 1938–2000*, Railmac Publications, SA, 2001, p. 22.

11 *RFDS of Australia Federal Council 50th Anniversary Yearbook*, (incorporating *Annual Report* and *Accounts* for the year ended 30 June 1986), p. 37.

15 Flying Intensive Care Units

1   Letter to author from Jack and Ruth Deakin, 3 January 2003.

2   *Airdoctor*, no. 222, September 2002, p. 5.

3   McPheat, pp. 49–50.

16 Sister Myra Blanch

1 Royal Flying Doctor Service of Australia, Federal Council, p. 237.
2 Bilton, p. 77.
3 *The Flying Doctor* (NSW Section), 1 April 1946, p. 23.
4 ibid, p. 24.
5 ibid, 1 July 1946, p. 44.
6 ibid, 1 January 1948, p. 4.
7 ibid, 1 July 1947, p. 54.
8 Royal Flying Doctor Service of Australia (NSW Section) booklet, p. 17.
9 *Australian Council of the RFDS of Australia Annual Report 2000*, p. 17.

17 No Place for a Woman

1 Flynn, *Northern Territory and Central Australia*, p. 9.
2 *The Inlander*, vol. 5, no. 2, 1918–19, p. 98.
3 ibid.
4 *Frontier News*, vol. 68, 1968, p. 12. Used with permission of Frontier Services.
5 *The NSW Presbyterian*, 8 April 1949, p. 15.
6 *The Presbyterian Messenger*, 16 October 1931, p. 252.
7 Bilton, p. 53.
8 *The Presbyterian Messenger*, 14 March 1930, p. 575.
9 Burchill, p. 39.
10 *The Presbyterian Messenger*, 16 October 1931, p. 252.
11 JC Finlayson, *Life and Journeyings in Central Australia*, 1925, (Melbourne: Arbuckle, Waddell), p. 52.
12 *The NSW Presbyterian*, 18 August 1932, p. 418.
13 Burchill, p. 67.
14 Janet Dickinson, *Jessie Litchfield: Grand Old Lady of the Territory*, Janet Dickinson, Blackwater, Qld, 1982, p. 96.
15 *The Presbyterian Messenger*, 1920, p. 352.
16 Arch Grant, *Camel Train & Aeroplane: The Story of Skipper Partridge*, Rigby, Adelaide, 1981, p. 126.
17 *The NSW Presbyterian*, 6 May 1949, p. 15.
18 ibid, 23 July 1948, p. 14.
19 Burchill, p. 141.
20 *The Flying Doctor* (NSW Section), 1 July 1948, p. 45.

18 Nurses in Full Flight

1 *The Presbyterian Messenger*, 28 June 1929, p. 875.
2 *The NSW Presbyterian*, 6 May 1945, p. 15.
3 *The NSW Presbyterian*, 11 February 1949, p. 12.
4 Bilton, p. 57.
5 ibid.
6 Jill Newlands, 'Neither invisible or forgotten: The RFDS nurses' story from the life and times of Myra Blanch, the first 'flying nurse', 1945–54', PhD thesis (submitted), Menzies School of Health Research, University of Sydney, 2003.
7 Royal Flying Doctor Service of Australia, Federal Council, p. 197.

8 *Australian Council of the RFDS of Australia Annual Report 2001*, p. 5.
9 'Standards for Flight Nursing Practice', Flight Nurses Australia website
   <http://isas.org.au/FNA/Home.htm>.

19 Early Remedies

1 Western Australian Centre for Rural and Remote Medicine website
   <http://www.wacrrm.uwa.edu.au/>.
2 Fysh, pp. 160–1.
3 *The Inlander*, vol. 19, 1927, pp. 74–5; *The Medical Journal of Australia*, 12 November 1927,
   p. 699.
4 *The NSW Presbyterian*, 1928, p. 638.
5 ibid, p. 766.
6 *The Inlander*, vol. 5, no. 2, 1918–19, p. 73.
7 Simpson, p. 50.
8 *The NSW Presbyterian*, 1929, p. 686.
9 *Sydney Morning Herald*, 6 February 1939, p. 5.
10 *The NSW Presbyterian*, 1929, p. 446.
11 Bill 'Swampy' Marsh, *Great Flying Doctor Stories*, ABC Books, Sydney, 1999, p. 126.
12 *The Flying Doctor* (NSW Section), 1 April 1941, p. 36.
13 *The Medical Journal of Australia*, 12 November 1927, p. 697.
14 *The Messenger*, 1921, p. 576.
15 Plowman, *The Man from Oodnadatta*, p. 190.
16 Myrtle Rose White, *No Roads Go By*, Rigby, Adelaide, 1932, p. 77.
17 ibid, p. 158.
18 *The Medical Journal of Australia*, 6 January 1951, p. 51.
19 Flynn, *The Bushman's Companion*, p. 6.
20 *The Inlander*, vol. 1, no. 1, 1913, p. 8.
21 ibid, p. 23.
22 Eve Pownall, *Australian Pioneer Women*, Viking O'Neill, Ringwood, Vic., 1988, p. 271.
23 White, p. 29.

20 Lifting the Burden

1 Burchill, p. 92.
2 *The NSW Presbyterian*, 1931, p. 14.
3 *The Medical Journal of Australia*, 31 March 1928, p. 410.
4 ibid, 1 February 1958, p. 131.
5 Burchill, p. 171.
6 Letter to author from Dr W Scott Kennedy, 23 January 2003.
7 ibid.
8 ibid.
9 Hudson, p. 48.
10 Timothy O'Leary, *Western Wings of Care: A Personal Memoir of Aviation Development and
   Clinical Life with the Royal Flying Doctor Service in Outback Australia*, Amphion Press,
   Brisbane, 1988, p. 37.

21 The Modern Approach

1 'Bases and Services', in *Australian Council of the RFDS Annual Report 2002*, p. 2.
2 ibid, 'Facts at a Glance', p. 1.
3 *Airdoctor*, May, 1999, p. 3.
4 *Australian Council of the RFDS Annual Report 2001*, p. 12.
5 'They Keep Us Flying', in *Australian Council of the RFDS Annual Report 2002*, p. 4.
6 *The Inlander*, vol. 20, 1929, p. 45.
7 Marsh, pp. 35–6.
8 Robin Miller, *Flying Nurse*, FA Thorpe (Publishing), Anstey, Leicestershire, 1979, pp. 390–1. (First published by Rigby, Adelaide, 1971)
9 *The South Eastern Flyer*, no. 2, 2001, p. 3.
10 Jill Newlands, 'Neither invisible or forgotten: The RFDS nurses' story from the life and times of Myra Blanch, the first "flying nurse", 1945–54', PhD thesis (submitted), Menzies School of Health Research, University of Sydney, 2003.

Bibliography

. . . .

Books

Affleck, Arthur H, *The Wandering Years*, Longmans, Green, Croydon, Vic., 1964.

Aplin, Graeme, Foster, SG, & McKernan, Michael, eds, *Australians: A Historical Dictionary*, Fairfax, Syme & Weldon Associates, Broadway, NSW, 1987.

Bilton, John, *The Royal Flying Doctor Service of Australia: Its Origin, Growth and Development*, Royal Flying Doctor Service of Australia, Federal Council, Sydney, 1961.

Brearley, Sir Norman, *Australian Aviator*, Rigby, Adelaide, 1971.

Burchill, Elizabeth, *Australian Nurses Since Nightingale 1860–1990*, Spectrum Publications, Richmond, Vic., 1992.

Burchill, Elizabeth, *Innamincka*, Rigby, Adelaide, 1960.

Cooter, Robert B, *The Air Doctors of South Australia: A Brief History of Medicine in Aero-medical Operations in South Australia, 1938–2000*, Railmac Publications, SA, 2001.

Copley, Greg, *Australians in the Air*, Rigby, Adelaide, 1976.

Dawson, Dr Len, *Skydoctor: Based on the Adventures and Experiences of a Flying Doctor in the 1950s*, Gypsy Publications, Wingham, NSW, 1995.

Dickinson, Janet, *Jessie Litchfield: Grand Old Lady of the Territory*, J. Dickinson, Blackwater, Qld, 1982.

Duguid, Charles, *Doctor and the Aborigines*, Rigby, Adelaide, 1972.

Farwell, George, *Down Argent Street: The Story of Broken Hill*, FH Johnston Publishing, Sydney, 1948.

Finlayson, JC, *Life and Journeyings in Central Australia*, 1925 (Melbourne: Arbuckle, Waddell).

Flynn, John, *The Bushman's Companion: A Handful of Hints for Outbackers*, Home Mission Committee of the Presbyterian Church of Victoria, Melbourne, 1910.

Flynn, John, *Northern Territory and Central Australia: A Call to the Church*, Angus & Robertson, Sydney, 1912.

Fysh, Sir Hudson, *Qantas Rising: The Autobiography of the Flying Fish / Sir Hudson Fysh*, Angus & Robertson, Sydney, 1965.

Grant, Arch, *Camel Train & Aeroplane: The Story of Skipper Partridge*, Rigby, Adelaide, 1981.

Griffiths, Max, *The Silent Heart: Flynn of the Inland*, Kangaroo Press, Kenthurst, NSW, 1993.

Gunn, Mrs Aeneas, *We of the Never-Never*, Angus & Robertson, North Ryde, NSW, 1905.

Harley, Jane F, *Mantle of Safety: The Flying Doctor Service*, Robert Hale, London, 1963.

Henry, Mona, *From City to the Sandhills of Birdsville*, Copyright Publishing, Qld, 1994.

Hill, Ernestine, *Flying Doctor Calling*, Angus & Robertson, Sydney, 1947.

Hill, Ernestine, *The Great Australian Loneliness*, Angus & Robertson, North Ryde, NSW, 1940.

Hudson, Harry, *Flynn's Flying Doctors*, The Specialty Press Ltd, Melbourne, 1956.

Idriess, Ion L, *Flynn of the Inland*, Angus & Robertson, Sydney, 1932.

Jensen, Peter R, *From the Wireless to the Web: The Evolution of Telecommunications 1901–2001*, University of New South Wales Press, Sydney, 2000.

King, Norma, *Wings over the Goldfields: The 50 Year History of the Eastern Goldfields Section of the RFDS of Australia*, RFDS (Eastern Goldfields Section) and Hesperian Press, Carlisle, WA, 1992.

Litchfield, J, *Far-North Memories*, Angus & Robertson, Sydney, 1930.

McKay, Fred, *Traeger: The Pedal Radio Man*, Boolarong Press, Moorooka, Qld, 1995.

McKenzie, Maisie, *Flynn's Last Camp*, Boolarong Publications, Brisbane, 1985.

McKenzie, Maisie, *Fred McKay: Successor to Flynn of the Inland*, Boolarong Publications, Brisbane, 1990.

McPheat, W Scott, *John Flynn: Apostle to the Inland*, Hodder & Stoughton, London, 1963.

Marsh, Bill 'Swampy', *Great Flying Doctor Stories*, ABC Books, Sydney, 1999.

Miller, Robin, *Flying Nurse*, FA Thorpe (Publishing), Anstey, Leicestershire, 1979. (First published by Rigby, Adelaide, 1971)

Miller, Robin, *Sugarbird Lady*, comp. & ed. Harold Dicks, Rigby, Adelaide, 1979.

O'Leary, Timothy, *North and Aloft: A Personal Memoir of Service and Adventure with the Royal Flying Doctor Service in Far Northern Australia*, Amphion Press, Brisbane, 1988.

O'Leary, Timothy, *Western Wings of Care: A Personal Memoir of Aviation Development and Clinical Life with the Royal Flying Doctor Service in Outback Australia*, Amphion Press, Brisbane, 1988.

Page, Michael, *The Flying Doctor Story 1928–78*, Rigby, Adelaide, 1977.

Plowman, RB, *The Boundary Rider*, Angus & Robertson, Sydney, 1935.

Plowman, RB, *The Man from Oodnadatta*, Angus & Robertson, Sydney, 1934.

Pownall, Eve, *Australian Pioneer Women*, Viking O'Neil, Ringwood, Vic., 1988.

Royal Flying Doctor Service of Australia, Federal Council, *Royal Flying Doctor Service of Australia: Australia's Unique Outback Medical Organisation*, Sydney, 1990.

Rudolph, Ivan, *Flynn's Outback Angels Vol. I: Casting the Mantle*, Central Queensland University Press (Outback Books), Rockhampton, Qld, 2001.

Rudolph, Ivan, *John Flynn: Of Flying Doctors and Frontier Faith*, Dove, North Blackburn, Vic., 1996.

Simpson, George, *Diary Letters of George Simpson: June, July, August 1927*, Australian Inland Mission, 1933.

White, Myrtle Rose, *No Roads Go By*, Rigby, Adelaide, 1932.

Wilson, George, *The Flying Doctor Story: A Pictorial History of the Royal Flying Doctor Service of Australia*, Magazine Art (Aust.), Hampton, Vic., 1989.

Woldendorp, Richard & McDonald, Roger, *Australia's Flying Doctors*, Pan Macmillan, Sydney, 1994.

Magazines/Journals

The Flying Doctor, 1940–1968, published by the NSW Section of the Australian Aerial Medical Services, later the Royal Flying Doctor Service.

Frontier News, 1932–1989, published by the Australian Inland Mission and later by its successor, the Uniting Church in Australia Frontier Services.

The Inlander, 1913–1929, published by the Australian Inland Mission.

The NSW Presbyterian, 1926–1965, official journal of the Presbyterian Church in New South Wales.

The Presbyterian Messenger, 1919–1965, official journal of the Presbyterian Church of Victoria and Tasmania.

Reports

Australian Council of the Royal Flying Doctor Service Annual Reports 1992–2002.

Barclay, J, 'The Royal Flying Doctor Service of Australia: The nurses' story', *Oral History Association of Australia Journal*, no. 20, 1988, pp. 52–8.

Collings, JW, *8000 Miles by Air Around Australia*, Report on a Tour of Inspection for the Federal Council of Australian Aerial Medical Services and Australian Aerial Medical Services (Victorian Section), June 1939.

Report of the Australian Inland Mission Board, September 1928.

Royal Flying Doctor Service of Australia Federal Council Annual Reports 1962, 1983, 1984, 1986.

Index

228

INDEX